Life in the Cave
The Series

LIFE in the
CAVE

THE SERIES

CELIA MARIE

Celia Marie, LLC
2020

Celia Marie, LLC

Published in the United States of America

ISBN: 978-1-71688-515-0
1. Health & Fitness/Diseases/Immune System
2. Health & Fitness/Diseases/General

For Mom and Papa

You are my heroes.
When I look at the brightest stars I know that you
are both smiling on me and encouraging me each step
of the way. Thank you for the beautiful dreams that
you both bring to me to keep us close. I love you both
so very much. I look forward to singing in Heaven's
choir with you when it's my time to join you both.
And, yes, Mom, there are many stars in your crown.
Thank you for teaching me about unconditional love,
forgiveness and reminding me to SMILE. And, Papa,
YOU are living proof that there are angels in Heaven.

BOOK ONE

Life in the Cave
Overcoming Graves' Disease

LIFE in the
CAVE

OVERCOMING GRAVES' DISEASE

CELIA MARIE

Celia Marie, LLC
2020

For Ri

You are everything to me and
you are God's mouthpiece in your generation.
I love you, Ri.

Joel 2:28

ACKNOWLEDGEMENTS

Pat--thank you for your financial support and for providing the much needed medical insurance. Malachi 3:10

Glynis--I could have never made it without you! Thank you for your love and for being there for my family during my surgery. Thanks for all of your prayers and the laughter! Proverbs 17:22

Pastor W. Donald and Betty Price, The Late Dr. John and Peg Howerton, Pastor Dan and Pamelia LaPaglia, Todd and Barbara Kane, Glynis Bonser, Debbie (Welch) Lowe, Richard Pollak and Garry Lowe--each of your prayers have been such a source of strength and encouragement for me and my family. I love all of you dearly and you all are like family to me. (Of course Dan and Pamelia are family!) Thank you for your belief that I would not die but live. Psalm 118:17

Eric--thank you! Jeremiah 29:11

FOREWORD

I confess to feeling apprehensive when Celia approached me about writing this entry. I immediately thought of a number of our mutual friends and acquaintances whom I believed to be more worthy and better assets to her offering. After relating this to her, Celia, in her normal grace, convinced me of the reasons that her finger pointed in my direction. So with her words clearly in my memory, I humbly pick up my pen and offer these words.

As a person who has also travelled the long road from illness to diagnosis and all of the avenues in between, I readily identified with Celia Marie's journey. In this journal of the beginning phases of a disease that has forever changed her life, Celia, exposes not only the confusion related to symptoms of early disease but has also outlined the influence of culture and spirituality upon the winding road from diagnosis to treatment...some of which kept her from seeking early assistance.

Life in the Cave is a story of Celia Marie's journey with Graves' disease, yet, I believe that anyone who has suffered through a chronic diagnosis will be able to see the mirror of recognition turned towards them.

Celia has crafted her story with honesty, sensitivity, and humility. She has seen a need and found a way to fill it. Due to lack of informational accounts from those living with this ailment, Celia stepped into the void to offer her story...her powerful, sad, yet hopeful story. With courage and optimism, she has laid her heart before you like a living sacrifice.

Although the book that you now hold in your hands chronicles my friend's journey with Graves' disease, if we are truly willing to reflect, I believe that like Celia Marie, we can all admit to being cave dwellers.

--Zayne Spencer
2009

INTRODUCTION

An Irish doctor, Robert James Graves, discovered Graves' disease in the 1830s. A decade later, German doctor Karl Adolph von Basedow reported the same symptoms as Dr. Grave. Europeans are more likely to be familiar with Basedow's disease which is the same as Graves' disease. I'm an American and, thus, will be referring to my formal diagnosis of Graves' disease throughout my journal.

Famous celebrities and public figures who have been diagnosed with Graves' disease include Joe Biel, George H.W. Bush, Barbara Bush, Toni Childs, Rodney Dangerfield, Bobby Engram, Marty Feldman, Diane Finley, Heino and Maggie Smith. The second president of the United States, John Adams, reportedly suffered from Graves' disease, too.

Graves' disease is a thyroid disorder caused by an autoimmune reaction. The trigger for the autoimmune reaction was still unknown at the time of this writing. Although Graves' disease is not curable, it is treatable.

I was compelled to write about my personal journey with Graves' disease because there was a lack of writings out there dealing with this unique disease. I believe that you're reading this journal because either you have been diagnosed with Graves' disease or someone that you love/know has been diagnosed with Graves' disease.

I want to share with you that I have written this journal in a very personal and transparent style. You will start with me before my formal diagnosis of Graves' disease and walk with me through the first two (2) years of my battle with Graves' disease until the night before my life would change forever. It is my deepest desire that you will receive relevant information that will encourage you and bring you hope.

CHAPTER
ONE

SPRING 2005

During the spring of 2005 I began to notice that I was losing a little bit of weight. I was very pleased. I had gained about twenty pounds for the past couple of years and it was very encouraging to have my clothes fit more loosely. I was beginning to get compliments on my slimmer body. What's not to love about that?

Two weeks later I noticed that I was getting tired earlier in the day than was normal. It was approaching the end of the school year. My pre-school class was getting spring fever. I figured that my antsy students' behavior may have been the reason that I was getting tired so much earlier. I really didn't think much about it after that.

We began preparing for the spring play and, as a result, we had to walk over to a different building than we were accustomed to for practice. The building was about an 1/8th of a mile from my classroom. By the end of the week I began having some trouble with pain in one of my legs. I figured that it would go away if I didn't put a whole lot of strain on it. The spring play came and went but the pain in my leg remained.

It was now the last week of school which was a very busy time of the school year. The end-of-year class party required a lot of preparation because I wanted to make it special for my students. The last day of school was always so bittersweet for me. I thought that I was doing a great job keeping it hidden just how fatigued I really was and how much the pain in my leg was increasing. *Maybe all I need is a week of relaxing*, I thought.

The week between the end of the school year and the beginning of the Sizzlin' Summer school program went by way too fast. Maria (my daughter) and I looked at each other in amazement--it was now time to begin the summer program at the school.

I was so thankful to be a teacher at the school that Maria attended. It was a blessing to have her help me get my class set up for the summer session. I tried so hard to not reveal to her how tired I was and how much my leg hurt. In fact, around 1:00 p.m. each day I would experience a wave of extreme exhaustion and develop a splitting headache at that hour. I thought, *If I just take it easy this summer hopefully the fatigue and pain in my leg will subside.*

During the first month of the Sizzlin' Summer school program I began to get my edge back. I was not as tired. I was very encouraged that I had more energy. I rationalized that the less demanding schedule was the reason that I was feeling better. Really though, in the back of my mind I had not totally convinced myself that all was well. I was still losing weight and not even trying. Although very grateful for the weight loss, I couldn't help wondering if something was wrong. I thought it had to be just my imagination. Besides, Pat (my husband) seemed especially happy to have a slimmer wife by his side!

The month of June and the first part of July went by fast. It was the middle of summer 2005 and I had lost even more weight. Now twenty pounds lighter, I was excited to be able to purchase even smaller size clothes. However, the pain in my leg was getting much worse and I was limping around most of the time. I thought that I had probably just pulled a muscle because I had been exercising. I decided that it would be wise for me to lighten up on the exercising; just until my leg stopped hurting so much.

By the end of summer 2005 my limping was so noticeable that Pastor W. Donald Price of Cathedral Christian Center in Glendale, Arizona asked me why I was limping. I had now lost forty pounds. Even though I was experiencing pain in my leg, I was proud to be so much thinner! My coworkers asked me if I was on a special diet and I told them, truthfully, no. I was receiving compliments all of the time on how good I looked since I had lost so much weight. I thought to myself, *I'd rather be thin even though I'm limping around.*

The Sizzlin' summer program was now over and it was the first week of August. I was participating in teacher in-service week. One of our in-service activities was a prayer walk over our campus. We would pray over each classroom. When we reached Maria's classroom, I sat down on the floor by Maria's desk. After our prayer for the students and teacher's upcoming school year, I attempted to stand up but my legs were so weak that I could not stand. I had to ask two coworkers to help me get back to my feet. Something was very wrong. I was starting to get scared. I did not know what was wrong but I did know that this was not normal for me. One of our buildings was two-story. Since I was still able to walk up and down the stairs I did not fully heed my body's warning that I needed to seek medical attention.

I stopped losing weight and the pain in my leg finally subsided. I thought that I must be getting better. The only issue that I was dealing with now was my fatigue. *Well, I am a teacher and it's the beginning of a new year*, I thought, *I must just need to give myself more time to adjust to the new school year.*

CHAPTER TWO

FALL 2005

Because September was full of school activities and meetings I always looked forward to a break from cooking in the hot kitchen and dinner at a restaurant instead.

It is hot, I thought, *Why am I always so hot?* It was now fall and I was still hot. It felt like it was 110 degrees even though in reality, it was a comfortable seventy-four degrees inside the restaurant.

I had also discovered that whenever I went out in the sun, my eyes would literally hurt. The sun appeared so bright that I would have to squint my eyes and even entirely shut them because the sun was so painful. This is why many Graves' disease sufferers wear dark sunglasses. That painful experience had never happened to me before. The sun was like a blinding light which hit my eyes with such force that it literally hurt.

I also noticed that my eyes were exceedingly red all of the time. I thought that they were red because I was fatigued most of the time. When you suffer from Graves' disease you are not just a little tired. You are perpetually wiped out. You wake up tired and you are tired all of the time you are awake. It is common to experience insomnia and your eyes are prone to redness due to lack of adequate sleep.

I came to the conclusion that I was a hypochondriac. I have a Bachelor's Degree in Science with a major in psychology. I told myself that I really needed to get over this obsessive behavior and thinking about my health issues constantly.

- - - - - - -

The new school year brought a full class roster. I went home exhausted at the end of each day. I was becoming more irritable during the day. I chalked it up to being overworked. Plus, I thought that with all the new students it would probably take awhile to get into a schedule.

Maria was in third grade now and she was such a blessing as she enthusiastically helped me any way she could. We enjoyed our drive to school together and she was adjusting well to the fact that we had to come to school a half-hour earlier than her classmates because I was required to attend daily staff devotions. I was so proud of my daughter for being so mature and handling being a staff kid so well.

I used to take the stairs up to our staff devotions room daily but my legs had become so weak that I now had to take the elevator daily. This was so devastating to me because I used to enjoy walking so much. *Little did I realize that the beginning of loss that I was to experience over the next two and a half years had started in the fall of 2005.*

CHAPTER
THREE

WINTER 2005

The first semester went by swiftly. Maria liked Mrs. Oakerman, her third grade teacher because she was consistently friendly and liked to joke with her. One day after school we went shopping for holiday outfits.

I was so very proud to be able to fit into size eight clothes again for the holiday season. I dismissed the questions that my co-workers were asking whether I was okay, and whether I thought I should see a doctor about my weight loss. In response, I thought, *No! I'm just happy to be near the weight that I used to be for so many years.*

I was getting used to the perpetual fatigue that I experienced daily. Around 1:00 p.m. each day I still became exhausted and had a splitting headache. At least after about a couple of hours the splitting headache would finally go away.

The holiday season was approaching and it was a joy to have Maria help me decorate my classroom for Christmas. We had so much fun making decorations, buying gifts for my students and creating their stockings. I love the holidays. I love the fact that secular radio stations play music about Jesus! The joy of the holiday season outweighed the concerns that I had in regards to my health issues. I chose to laugh and enjoy the holiday season with my daughter. We worked hard to prepare for my class Christmas party and it was a huge success. I was so proud of the way that Maria interacted with my students. I enjoyed serving my students during the joyous holiday season. I bought each of them a small snow globe that fit perfectly in their tiny hands.

Maria and I enjoyed our Christmas break. It was such a blessing to bake Christmas cookies and desserts together because Maria and I were always busy with all of the school-related activities most of the time. We welcomed opportunities to relax and spend part of our day doing fun activities together. On Christmas Eve day I prepared our traditional homemade lasagna (my spouse says that he married me because I bake amazing lasagna) along with Christmas Eve Cake (Torte Vigilia di Natale). Although Pat had to work on Christmas Eve and was tired while we ate our dinner we still enjoyed the tradition of our homemade lasagna dinner as opposed to going out to a restaurant. Although I was weak and had to buy pre-shredded mozzarella cheese and pre-diced onions I still boiled the lasagna pasta myself and prepared the homemade sauce. After we ate, I enjoyed playing Christmas carols and holiday music on the piano for my family. Each day was such a joy because I could relax and have fun. *I refused to dwell on how fatigued I was despite all the relaxing that I was doing--it just didn't make sense to be constantly fatigued and I just wanted to focus on the joy of the season.*

I continued to experience the splitting headaches around 1:00 p.m. each day every afternoon. Towards the end of Christmas break I became ill with walking pneumonia. It was horrible to be so ill. The antibiotics were not working and my 104 degree temperature wouldn't go away. I had to have my doctor prescribe a stronger antibiotic. I was miserable. I went to the doctor and discovered that I had walking pneumonia. He prescribed an antibiotic but after taking the full ten days prescription I was still running a high fever. He prescribed a stronger antibiotic. It isn't unusual to contract communicable illnesses when working with young children. I didn't link the walking pneumonia with the fatigue I was feeling because my doctor shared that walking pneumonia had been going around during the holidays that year.

It was now 2006 and we had a nice Valentine's Day (we called it Senior Friend Day because we honored the seniors in our families and extended family/close friends) party at the school. Once again, my daughter helped me set up my classroom for the party. We made special valentines for each student. C.J.'s (a student of mine) amazing mom, Kelly, organized the special Valentine craft projects. She was a Godsend. I always looked forward to seeing Kelly; she was so balanced and always a pleasure to interact with. Rochelle (her sweet and cheerful son Joshua was in my class) was a very supportive parent who had organized our class Harvest party during the fall semester. Glynette, my student Tiffany's mom, was quick to offer an encouraging word to me and we would often laugh together. Glynette treated me with a lot of respect and kindness; I treasured my friendship with Glynette. These are examples of a few of my very supportive parents. I thanked God for them.

SPRING 2006

I made it through the Parent Teacher conferences even though it was so exhausting preparing for them. I cannot believe that I had such a big class. I was so thankful that the Lord gave me strength to get through each day despite the ever increasing fatigue. I was also beginning to notice that I had to use the restroom more often. I thought I was just drinking too much water. Even one of my coworkers commented on how much more often I was using the restroom. We joked about it but this was just one more cause for concern that I began to ponder.

Beginning in March of 2006 I started falling asleep at work. My students would laugh and Tiffany, one of my outgoing students, would say "Teacher, wake up!" as she giggled.

I noticed that my hair was beginning to fall out. I also observed that my neck area was slightly swollen. Sandy and June, my coworkers, noticed the swelling, too. Even though I knew in my heart of hearts that something was wrong, I still was trying to dismiss all of these observances as hypochondria. In retrospect, I believe that I continually dismissed my symptoms because I was so very frightened that once I saw a doctor the diagnosis was going to be very serious. I was just not ready to emotionally deal with whatever my medical condition was.

One day my boss came into my classroom and said, "You are anxious, aren't you?" It was all starting to fall apart. I couldn't hide the symptoms any longer because they were beginning to be noticeable by others. I didn't know what to do. I loved teaching. I loved being with my students. I loved their excitement and wonder at the world they were discovering. I enjoyed having Maria come into my classroom at the end of the day. Sometimes she brought one of her friends with her.

I had been teaching since the spring of 2000 at the school, and, as a result, my daughter and I had practically lived there for the past six years. I believe that deep down I knew that my days at the school were coming to a close. I was getting scared.

We were once again approaching the end of another school year. I was so exhausted that I was actually relieved that the school year was almost over. Maria helped me plan the end-of-year school party. I didn't do as much as I had done in the past. I was just too fatigued. I was thankful that

Kayden's (my soft-spoken student) mom, Angela, helped with the party. She was another very supportive parent.

Maria and I had our week-long break before the Sizzlin' Summer school program began. I was exhausted that whole week at home and was not physically, mentally or emotionally ready to come back for the school's summer program. By this time I could no longer hide my illness from my husband, Pat. He noticed that something was wrong. I told him that I just could no longer work at the school. He agreed. He was excited because he thought I would have time to be his loan officer for his real estate clients. *Neither one of us realized that I was only going to get much, much worse.*

On June 9, 2006 I turned in my resignation. It was one of the most painful days in my life. My friend, Carla, really helped me get through that day. I was an emotional wreck. I remember crying as I told Glynette that I was quitting. I had known Glynette for the past two years because two of her older daughters whom I dearly loved had also been in my pre-school class.

My daughter helped me pack up all of my teaching supplies. My Buick Skylark was totally full of over six years worth of teaching supplies along with gifts that I had received from students and coworkers. As we drove away with tears in our eyes we struggled to grasp the reality that we would never be coming back to Cathedral Christian Academy.

CHAPTER
FOUR

SUMMER 2006

Now that I was officially unemployed, I started sleeping later and later in the mornings. I thought I was just catching up on rest. Pat would go to work in the mornings and come home to the same dirty dishes on the dining room table that were there when he had left for work earlier that day. I was getting to the point where I just did not have the strength to do the smallest of tasks. Our home was more and more cluttered. I could not keep up with the daily chores. Pat was not only working full time along with working on real estate transactions, he was also starting to do the household chores. He didn't realize that I literally could not do the chores. I was so exhausted. I didn't have any strength. In fact I was so weak that I could no longer get up from sitting down without having to hold on to something for support.

Not only did I observe that I was sleeping more and more and becoming even weaker, I was now losing actual clumps of hair instead just strands of hair like I had in the past.

It was heartbreaking because my hair used to be so long, thick and naturally wavy. I would cry when I brushed my hair because handfuls would come out. I was so frightened.

The summer was over and it was our wedding anniversary weekend. We decided to go to Flagstaff to celebrate (Flagstaff is where we went on our honeymoon eleven years prior). While we were in Flagstaff we decided to drive up to Williams where my brother lives.

We went to visit my brother and sister-in-law during early September. My brother observed that I was very nervous, had lost a lot of hair and weight, and could barely walk--he told me to go see a doctor right away. He later shared with me that my appearance that day was such that I looked as if I had aged twenty to thirty years since he last saw me.

A few days after visiting my brother I was asked to play a grand piano at a college restaurant on an ongoing basis. I accepted the gig and didn't anticipate any problems because I had been playing the piano for thirty-eight years. One day as I began to play my set I looked at the musical notes in front of me and had no idea what they were. I was very frightened. "What is happening to me?" I asked myself. On the way home from one of my piano playing sessions, I started scratching my eyelid because my eye felt gritty. We stopped at a store and my husband noticed that my eye was all bloody on the eyeball. It also appeared that my eyes had a frightened look and were slightly protruding. It was at this point that I knew that I had to see a doctor. Pat was scared that I might have an aneurysm. I believe that it was at this point that he finally realized he had a seriously ill wife who needed medical attention immediately.

I was able to see my family doctor the very next morning. I shared with him all of my symptoms. He had his nurse immediately draw my blood. My heart rate was 125 bpm. The normal heart rate is between 60-100 bpm. My blood test results came back as critical toxic. My doctor told me that he believed I was suffering from hyperthyroidism and Graves' disease. He prescribed Propranolol, a beta blocker which is a drug used to reduce the heart rate, and Methimazole, an anti-thyroid medication.

The function of the thyroid is to take iodine and convert it into thyroid hormones which affect nearly all tissues of the body regulating the body's metabolism. In fact, the thyroid's function is critical because it keeps the body's metabolism from over or under working.

The following morning I received a call from my doctor's office. I was to have a thyroid scan uptake within seventy-two hours and an ultrasound during the following week because he wanted to determine what the problem was with my thyroid. He didn't say what he was anticipating finding.

I was so scared. By now I needed assistance getting in and out of the car. I walked very slowly. I needed help lifting my legs from the parking lot to the actual sidewalk. I was very confused. My hands trembled so much that I could no longer write legibly. I could not focus. I was a mess. *What if I have thyroid cancer?* I thought.

CHAPTER
FIVE

During the month of October 2006, the thyroid scan and ultrasound were performed. The thyroid scan uptake was a two-day process. I was so frightened to have this test administered. I again asked myself, "what if I have thyroid cancer?" A few days after the thyroid scan uptake, I went to another center for the ultrasound. Based on the results of these tests, I was officially diagnosed with Hyperthyroidism and Graves' disease.

I met with Dr. Richard Dolinar, my thyroid specialist, weekly. He informed me that I could no longer drive an automobile until we could get my body stabilized and my confusion subsided. I was also to refrain from exercising; it was just too dangerous to attempt to exercise in my fragile, unstable physical condition.

My heart rate was still around 130 bpm---this was an alarming rate. The threat of congestive heart failure was staring me in the face. The thought of death was very real to me. I did not want to lose my nine year old daughter. I did not want Maria to experience the loss of her mother. She was too precious to me for me to give up on life. She was my life.

During this time, I was attempting to homeschool Maria, which was a very daunting task. We were utilizing the A Beka Academy DVD curriculum (A Beka was the curriculum that my daughter studied at Cathedral Christian Academy and the curriculum that I had used with my classes). Although the lesson plans were prepared for me, it was still difficult to keep up with her lessons.

I was getting weaker and weaker. I finally had to call A Beka Academy and explain how very ill I was. I asked for an extension for my daughter because we were so behind in her schoolwork. It was granted. Praise God! I was very thankful that A Beka Academy granted the extension for Maria's schoolwork.

My eyesight was also affected. I would see ripples (like the rippling water of a stream) in front of me. It lasted for several minutes. I never knew when this would occur. It was now getting to the point where I had trouble reading.

Pat continued to work full time, work on real estate deals when he wasn't at his full time job, and keep up with the household chores. It hurt me to watch him struggle with all of these responsibilities. I could see that the strain of all of the pressure was getting to him. I felt like such a failure. I saw the fear in Maria's eyes and that hurt me so much, too. My life was becoming so painful to live. Not only was I in physical, emotional and mental pain; Maria and Pat were experiencing pain too. "Why are we going through all of this suffering?" I lamented. The hardest part was to watch their pain and to feel so hopeless and helpless in helping them heal because my illness was the source of their pain. I wanted to make their pain go away so that they could take the shackles off of them that my Graves' disease was causing so they could be free of the "what if's"--especially for Maria. Maria and I have always been close. She is my only child. My pregnancy with Maria was high-risk; there was even a period when I was on bed rest. We are literally together 24/7. I can count on one hand the times that Maria was left with a babysitter and the babysitter was a family member.

Throughout Maria's life she has even slept with me on several occasions at night. In fact, when I first started seeing Dr. Dolinar Maria began sleeping with me again at night. We have never been self-conscious about public displays of affection. We're comfortable holding hands, kissing and embracing in front of others.

During November, I began to receive encouraging e-mails from Pastor W. Donald and Betty Price. They were my pastors for several years and have shown tremendous support and love to me and my family for over 20 years. They shared that they were taking "a stand for miracles to become evident because we are trusting and believing in (His) word." As I read their e-mail around midnight, the presence of God came into my home office in a mighty way. I responded to their email with "Yes, He is our Healer and Miracle Maker-- oh, how I believe that completely." I had also begun to read twenty-four Bible verses daily dealing specifically with healing.

During mid-November, I met with Dr. Dolinar and he informed me that it was time to schedule the Radioactive Iodine (RAI) treatment. November 19, 2006 was the day I was to go to the hospital for this treatment. A few days before the treatment I needed to begin taking steroids in an effort to keep my eyes from continuing to bulge after I stopped taking Methimazole, the anti thyroid medication.

I chose the Radioactive Iodine treatment over the Thyroidectomy option because the treatment was less invasive than surgery and I was so very frightened to go under the knife. The thought of a surgeon slitting near my vocal chords was not what I wanted to experience—I loved to sing and didn't want to have any damage done that would change or ruin my voice.

It was the evening before I was to go to the hospital for the Radioactive Iodine (RAI) treatment. I needed to make sure that I had everything ready for my return home. I was to be quarantined for awhile. I couldn't be in too close of proximity to others for a few days. I had to use special eating and drinking utensils. I had to sanitize the areas that I used before others could enter the area.

It was very difficult for me to accept that I would not be able to hug and kiss Maria for a while. We had always been affectionate with each other. I enjoy giving Maria a quick hug or kiss as a way of affirming her. I like to be physically close to her and I didn't like that opportunity to be taken away. I would never again take for granted the freedom to be physically close to Maria.

Before I went to sleep I prayed, "*Father God, please go before me. Please be with each medical staff personnel who will be part of this RAI treatment. Please let this treatment be effective and heal me of Graves' disease and Hyperthyroidism. Please take away my daughter's, my husband's and my fear. Please help me to relax so that I can get some sleep tonight. In Jesus' name I pray, Amen.*"

CHAPTER SIX

On the drive to the hospital I could definitely feel the prayers of intercessors for me. Their prayers helped me to stay calm and peaceful. Maria went with me to the hospital. We spent over an hour waiting to be called. Then we met with the technician. He discovered that a required blood test had not been administered. This meant that I had to go to the basement of the hospital to get my blood drawn. We then waited nearly two hours to receive the results of that required blood test. By now we had been at the hospital for nearly four (4) hours. I finally was called in for the RAI treatment. The actual treatment didn't take long at all. We all joked about how I would be glowing now that I had taken the radioactive capsules!

I was so relieved to be going home. I was so excited that this treatment was going to stop my overactive thyroid, my bulging eyes would shrink back to their normal size and I wouldn't have to take the beta blockers anymore. *I thanked God for modern medicine. It will be nice to get my energy back for the Christmas holidays*, I thought.

About a week before Christmas my whole family was ill. We went to the doctor and were all diagnosed with walking pneumonia. Since the doctor told us that it was going around I did not connect that it could be something more serious causing my immune system to be weakened. We spent Christmas at home and concentrated on healing. This was the second Christmas in a row that I had been ill with walking pneumonia. Because we were contagious we discouraged family and friends from visiting. It was a disappointment to not be able to join in on the holiday festivities. *Little did I realize at the time what a huge disappointment the RAI treatment was going to prove.*

I continued to see Dr. Dolinar monthly. The anti thyroid medication helped my body gain the weight back that I should have been at for my height and body type. I no longer had weight loss issues; in fact, I was now two dress sizes bigger much to my chagrin. My thyroid levels improved a little which was great. However, I was starting to have more complications with my eyes. Dr. Dolinar recommended that I see an ophthalmologist. Graves' disease not only affects the eyesight but the actual structure of the eye area. It is common for the muscles around the eye to begin to swell (just like the swelling of the neck area due to the goiter--enlarged thyroid) when you have Graves' disease.

LATER WINTER 2006/WINTER 2007

I was still very fatigued. I now was experiencing major issues with insomnia. I also had horrible nightmares. Everything was working against me--I was afraid to go to sleep because of the nightmares but I was also so exhausted that I couldn't help but fall asleep. Then, I would wake up as soon as I reached a deeper phase of sleep due to the nightmares. It was a very frustrating and frightening cycle to go through every night.

I still experienced confusion and lack of focus. I gave up reading and watching movies because I just could not concentrate for more than a few minutes at a time. Confusion and lack of focus are common symptoms of Graves' disease sufferers.

I had reverted back to my old ways of not revealing to my family how truly awful I felt. On December 28, 2006 my mother-in-law, Carole, had been diagnosed with Stage 4 lung cancer. A few weeks after she was officially diagnosed with cancer, I offered to help her. She was trying so hard to be brave and strong. It was a very humbling time for both of us because we were both so ill yet trying to support each other. My heart broke watching the demise of her health. I was so scared wondering what would happen if I had thyroid cancer. I saw how much pain that she was in and it frightened me so much to see such a strong and courageous woman fighting for life and losing.

I did the best that I could while taking Carole to her doctor appointments and administering her meds. This was a sobering time for us. Maria was with us while I attempted to take care of my mother-in-law. She was so scared that her grammy was going to die. I knew that she was also scared that her mommy was going to die. It hurt me to see my nine year old daughter experiencing so much stress and fear. I felt so helpless.

It was now my forty-fourth birthday. I had lost a lot of hair. I was very depressed. A young woman at church told my husband that I looked "scary". Her comment really hurt me because I used to be attractive. I just wanted to die. Then I remembered my beautiful daughter, Maria, and I thought of the times in my life when I had to make the choice to live. When I was born the doctors told my parents that I had cerebral palsy, one of my legs was shorter than the other which would cause me to walk with a noticeable limp, and my eyesight was so damaged that I would eventually become blind. I proved the doctors wrong and never grew into any of those 'labels'. My parents provided the best care for me and through corrective eye surgery and several years of concentrated eye care I no longer needed to wear glasses.

Years later as an adult, once again I was faced with the choice to live. I wanted to see Maria grow up. I wanted to be at her high school graduation. I wanted to see her walk down the aisle on her wedding day. I wanted to share my life with her future children and enjoy watching them grow up. Now that I was a mom I chose desperately to live to watch my daughter "become." I wanted to share my thoughts with her on the choice to live and see if she had similar beliefs or if she would carve her own way. Choosing to live is one of the bravest choices one can ever make. I could not allow myself to give up on life even though, at that moment, I was just so exhausted and so broken; I was broken physically, emotionally, mentally, and spiritually. At this point, I stopped reading the twenty-four healing verses daily. I stopped going to church. I didn't even feel like praying anymore. In retrospect, I believe it was at this breaking point I subconsciously chose to live even though I halted my spiritual nourishment.

I remember the fear in Maria's eyes as we celebrated my birthday. I told her that everything would be okay. I assured her that I was not doing to die. We hugged and cried together. Knowing that Maria was suffering and fearful made me angry. As a mom, I wanted to protect her from all the bad of the world. I was a complete failure. I felt so sorry for my husband. The attractive woman that he married years earlier was gone. I was even ugly on the inside. I had lost hope. I began to believe that I wasn't going to be healed. I felt so lost. *It was during this winter season that I began to experience the first stirrings of what I would later refer to as life in the cave. I was aware that life was going on around me but for me time stood still. I was trapped in the prison of disease watching others (they were like shadows) going about their lives. They were going to work, going to the grocery store, going to church and going to the movies as I sat chained and motionless. I could see the light of life in a very far distance but directly all around me was darkness. I saw the outline of steps leading to a tall, locked gate far off in front of me and beyond that gate there were steps leading higher to the light. I often wondered if I would ever make it to the light and beyond.*

CHAPTER SEVEN

Carole was getting worse. The family called in a formal nurse to take care of her. I was relieved because I was in no shape to take care of her; plus, Maria was negatively affected by being around seriously ill loved ones. Maria was sad and scared most of the time and she would often cry. She would tell me that she didn't want me to die and hold on to me for dear life.

Although this winter season had begun to descend upon me, I still was reaching out to a friend of a friend. I had learned (while reading a post on the 77s, a Sacramento-based band, listserv) that Jan Volz was requesting prayer for Eric (his son) because he had been wrongfully accused of murder. In 2000, I had formed a prayer group and I asked my prayer group to pray for Jan's son, Eric. Jan added me to his master e-mail group and faithfully gave updates on Eric's situation. Eric had been falsely accused of murdering his ex-girlfriend, Doris Jimenez, on November 21, 2006 and he was still sitting in a jail in Nicaragua more than a month after his arrest. Eric's family was doing everything possible to get him back to the United States but the Nicaraguan authorities refused to release Eric. Not only was I scared for Carole's losing battle with cancer and my possible prognosis of thyroid cancer--I was also very scared for Eric. I had no idea, at the time, that it would take approximately another year for Eric to be released from prison.

On February 21, 2007 Eric Volz was sentenced to thirty years in prison--Nicaragua's maximum sentence. Eric, falsely accused, was suffering the gravest of injustices and inhumane treatment. This totally devastated me to know how much pain

Eric, his dad, his mom, his sister and loved ones were experiencing. My family had gone through a similar situation six years earlier, thus, I had so much empathy for the Volz and Anthony families. Eric's horrific situation was the catalyst for me to begin praying again. Another reason Eric's story caught my attention was because since I was a child I wanted to drive on the Pan American Highway through Nicaragua, Costa Rica and on to see the Panama Canal. To learn that Eric was being tortured in Nicaragua touched a personal chord of interest. I knew that the only way that I could help the Volz and Anthony families was to pray. Even though I did not believe in a miracle for myself I knew that God could open those prison doors for Eric just like He had for Paul and Silas. I was very uninhibited in my prayers for Eric's freedom. I was also praying for Doris' family and specifically for justice for Doris and that her true murderers would be revealed and apprehended. The prayers were also being lifted up for Maria. As the days turned into weeks and then into months I discovered that I was actively involved in daily prayer again.

Two days after Eric's sentencing, on February 23, 2007 Carole lost her battle with lung cancer. I wrote this to my prayer group: "This morning as I held Carole's hand she began to cross over the Jordan River--at approximately 11:40 a.m. she made it to the other side." I truly loved her. Not only had I lost my mother-in-law, I had lost my sister in the Lord. I would never hear her say "God bless" nor "how's my Celia?" and I would never experience the warmth of her hugs again. *Carole's death would officially begin my experience with life in the cave for the next eighteen months.*

CHAPTER EIGHT

SPRING 2007

Today, March 13, was my daughter's tenth birthday. We had a pizza party and celebrated with a Carvel cake. I enjoyed watching Maria laugh and play with her best friend Tabitha on her special day. For the last nine months Maria had worn such a sorrowful countenance and it warmed my heart to see her smile, giggle and chuckle for hours that day with Tabitha.

The day after her birthday, Maria was crying. I asked her what was wrong and she replied, "I miss Grammy. I wish that Grammy could have been here for my birthday." I knew my daughter was missing the special tradition she normally shared with her grandmother. They would spend time together, just them, usually going to lunch and then to Toys R Us. I knew that this had been terribly special to Maria, and now all I could do was give her a big hug and hold her until her sobs subsided.

About a week after her birthday, my husband took Maria and Tabitha to the humane society. They fell in love with an Australian Cattle Dog, christened Boomer at the humane society, and brought him home. Boomer was a wonderful new addition to the family. He was so well-behaved and very gentle. Boomer was tri-colored with the majority of his body black. His face looks like a beagle's and he has a white Bentley stripe above his nose. His black tail has a white tip. Boomer never jumped on a person and he never begged for food. The moment I looked into Boomer's beautiful brown eyes I fell in love with him. That night he chose to sleep right beside me on the floor and he still sleeps right beside me on his very own leather bed!

A few days after Boomer came to live with us we noticed that he had nightmares. We would gently wake him up and reassure him that he was okay, we loved him and would not hurt him. We would tell him that he was safe now.

Boomer often experienced his nightmares at the same times I was up with anxiety attacks. We were some pair. I finally just had to keep the TV on a Christian TV station all night long so that when I woke up with an anxiety attack I could calm myself down more easily. Once I awoke I rarely ever went back to sleep.

Due to the lack of sleep, I was also extremely irritable all of the time which put an incredible strain on my family. Further, Dr. Dolinar shared with us that it is common for several married Graves' disease sufferers to divorce because the personality of the Graves' disease sufferer tremendously alters and perpetual irritability is a common symptom. In fact in some marriages it is too difficult for the healthy partner to adjust to the personality (emotional and mental) changes that occur in the Graves' disease sufferer.

Pat continued to work long hours through the month of June while Maria and I daily conducted open houses at a property Pat had listed. Meanwhile, our house remained cluttered and the daily tasks continued to exhaust me. I was becoming more and more anxious as each day seemed to drag on with more clutter, more fatigue and more financial stress.

Dr. Dolinar checked my blood levels and discovered that my thyroid levels were sky-high again when I saw him in June for my regular three-month appointment. My pulse was also rapid. He prescribed Methimazole once again. I didn't like taking the Methimazole because it made me gain weight but I noticed I wasn't as anxious when I took the Methimazole so I began taking it again. He also increased my dosage of

Propranolol, the beta blocker. He told me that if I continued to feel anxious he would prescribe an anti-anxiety med for me.

My husband was planning a trip to Bushnell, Illinois for the annual Cornerstone Music Festival during the last days of June and first days of July. He hadn't been able to attend for several years and he wanted to take us for a family vacation along with his best friend's family of six. I did not want to go to Cornerstone because I was still feeling weak, confused, fatigued and anxious. Dr. Dolinar advised me not to go. I explained to him that this was a very special event that Pat rarely attended so Dr. Dolinar prescribed an anti-anxiety med and told me to call him any time on the trip if I needed to talk to him. *I never took the anti-anxiety med because I was too scared of the side effects that it could have on me.*

CHAPTER
NINE

SUMMER 2007

On the last Sunday of June 2007 we all loaded up in the RV and headed out for Cornerstone. We had six blowouts before we ever made it out of our home state. I was already a nervous wreck but I told Pat that I would go with him if he really wanted me to, so it was now Cornerstone or Bust!

We stayed at KOA Kampgrounds. I had never been RVing in my life. If I hadn't been so ill, I believe that I really would have enjoyed the experience more. We were supposed to arrive at Cornerstone on Wednesday morning but because of the issues with the tires we wound up arriving during the late afternoon on Thursday. I was already very irritated because I missed several of the bands that I wanted to see. I remember changing clothes in the RV and rushing (as best as I could because I was still very weak) to see Leigh Nash of Sixpence None the Richer. I got there just in time to hear her sing two songs before the end of her set.

Because I was so weak, Pat rented a golf cart for us so that we could get around the huge festival grounds. I spent each day at the Gallery Tent. There were a few bands playing there that I liked. I was content although my perpetual exhaustion put a damper on my happiness.

Sunday morning came way too fast and it was time to leave. Literally minutes before we left Cornerstone, Zayne (an internet friend whom I had never personally met) knocked on our RV door. Zayne told me that she vowed she wasn't going to leave Cornerstone until we finally got to meet in person. It was such a joy to spend about twenty minutes visiting with

Zayne. We had been internet friends for about three years when we connected on the 77s listserv. We were fans of other musical artists and bands, too. Over the years we shared bits and pieces of our lives through e-mail and discovered that we are both cat lovers.

After our visit we started down that dusty Cornerstone road to return home. It took us three days to drive back to Arizona. I was exhausted and so grateful to be home again. We had really missed our pets because Cornerstone wouldn't allow us to bring our pets. We arrived home on the fourth of July and I was exceedingly exhausted because we had been on the road in the RV for three consecutive days. When we walked in the house I was relieved and immediately stressed due to the total chaos of cluttering the house with two weeks of dirty laundry, bedding and camping equipment which were literally dumped in the living room, dining room and kitchen area. My husband took Maria to see the fireworks with friends so that she wouldn't miss out on the holiday festivities. After they left I went to bed totally exhausted and exasperated because of the clutter.

During the remainder of the summer I continued to have regularly scheduled appointments with Dr. Dolinar. He would measure my goiter and my eyes to see how far they had protruded in comparison with the previous visit. There was no change in the measurements. I was still struggling with anxiety attacks but they weren't as frequent as they had been in the past.

I was starting to feel a little normal in that I wasn't as tired and anxious and had even lost a couple of pounds. Dr. Dolinar reduced the dosage of my meds. My levels seemed to be holding on their own. It looked like the RAI treatment had finally taken.

I saw Dr. Dolinar in September of 2007 and he said that he wanted to see me again in December. I believe that I was still in denial during this time period. I had convinced myself that the goiter was shrinking and that my eyes weren't protruding as much. I was expecting to be told that he wouldn't want to see me for at least six months when I saw him in December. *I had no idea just how wrong I was.*

In November, Maria and I began making plans for our Thanksgiving meal. We decided that we wanted to spend Thanksgiving at a KOA Kampground. Maria and Pat worked very hard to get everything together for our Thanksgiving excursion.

Our neighbors at the KOA were from Australia. They had two teenage sons. We loved their Aussie accents. Our dog, Boomer, loved the extra attention from our neighbors. The weather was very pleasant and we had an enjoyable time on our Thanksgiving holiday. I enjoyed Maria and Pat tell of the fun experiences they had while riding in the go-cart on the hiking and go-cart trails. Boomer stayed at the campsite with me and we rested. After we rested I took him for a little walk around the KOA Kampground and up a small hiking trail.

Maria and Pat bought our Christmas tree during Thanksgiving weekend. They chose a big, beautiful fragrant Christmas tree. We were all so excited this holiday season. Our home was filled with the delicious aromas and scents of the seasons that resulted from our holiday baking. We were all extremely excited about it being Boomer's first Christmas. He appeared to sense the joy and wonder of the season, too. We had noticed that he wasn't having as many nightmares as he used to. Boomer was finally settling in. He was even gaining weight and I was gaining weight right along with him.

I went in for my December thyroid appointment. The appointment didn't last too long. Dr. Dolinar told me he wanted me to get my blood drawn that day. He said that there was no change in the measurement of my goiter and eyes. Dr. Dolinar informed me that he would call me with the results of my blood test. We wished each other a happy holiday season. I was certain that the next time I would see him again would probably be in around four to six months. *Little did I know that I would never see him again.*

CHAPTER
TEN

EARLY WINTER 2007

The phone rang and Dr. Dolinar's voice came on the answering machine. I walked over to pick up the phone. He told me the results of my blood tests. He went on to say that he could no longer help me. He referred me to his colleague, Dr. Daniel Duick, who handled the "tough" thyroid cases. I started to cry and thanked Dr. Dolinar for all that he had done for me. Once again I was scared. I was going to have to start all over again. I worried about whether I would like my new specialist, and whether I would be able to trust him with my life.

It was now Christmas Eve and I prepared my annual lasagna along with the Christmas Eve Cake (Torte Vigilia di Natale). On Christmas day we had Dijon Maple Spiral Sliced Ham with all of the holiday sides and pies for dessert. My family had been enjoying this Christmas meal for a few years and I didn't want them to miss out just because I was weak. The dinner was strained because I was exhausted, Pat was stressing out about finances and Maria was hurt that we were not having a festive atmosphere at the holiday table.

LATE WINTER 2008

On January 7, 2008 I met with my new thyroid specialist, Dr. Daniel Duick. He was very thorough; he personally performed my ultrasound. I was immediately impressed with him. He told me that he wanted to meet with me the following week to discuss our plan of action. When Dr. Duick and I met he informed me that I needed a total thyroidectomy because my goiter was huge and toxic. He said that he was surprised that I had lasted as long as I had. I was in very bad shape and was only going to get worse unless I got that toxic goiter removed from my body. He referred me to a surgeon: Dr. Richard Harding. I agreed to the surgery but I was terrified to go under the knife.

The following week I met with the surgeons, Dr. Harding and Dr. Bryce. They were young men; I had to choose whether I trusted them with my life. As my daughter and I drove away from their office, she started to cry. Maria said "Mommy, I don't want you to die." I told her that Dr. Harding and Dr. Bryce were excellent surgeons and they were going to help me get well. It was at that point that I chose to believe that I was in good hands.

My total thyroidectomy was scheduled for February 25, 2008. I had chosen the surgery to take place at a hospital very near my home.

Each day was very hectic as I tried to get everything in order for my surgery. There were a million little things to do that were all important. I was still very frightened to go under the knife. I had requested that several people, in addition to my prayer group, pray for me. An internet friend who became a great source of encouragement during this time was Marti. She was a diligent prayer warrior for myself and my family. Thank you, Marti!

I was having trouble sleeping at night because I was so frightened that I was going to die during the surgery. I tried to calm down. At times I actually did calm down for the sake of Maria because she was so frightened. I believe that the prayers that were being offered up for my family helped calm us. Many times we could sense the presence of the Lord with us.

On February 14 my daughter and my spouse brought home a beautiful, young bunny rabbit. I was very upset and irritable that they brought home a new pet so close to my surgery date; I didn't want to take the time to care for a new pet while trying to get ready for my upcoming surgery. I had to admit, though, that the bunny was adorable. It took a while for Maria to name her bunny. She finally decided to call him Snickers. Snickers enchanted us all with his winning ways. He became the perfect pet. Although Snickers could not verbally communicate, he was a very effective non-verbal communicator. He would hop excitedly to the refrigerator when I opened the door to give him a carrot, lettuce or a strawberry. Then he would perform a bunny spin in jubilation of his edible treat. He would also eagerly wiggle his nose in anticipation of his favorite foods. He was so adorable when he did his flopsies. As he grew older his markings turned sable and his fur was very soft. He was also quite curious. He thought that the telephone, computer, stereo and television cables and wires were roots. Although Snickers was just a small bunny, he brought so much light into my dark days. *At the time, I did not realize how therapeutic Snickers was going to be for me during the next nine months.*

It was now eleven days before my surgery and I still hadn't drawn up a will. I needed to make sure there were funds in the bank account to cover my insurance co-pay for the surgery. I was dragging my feet. I was scared. My friend, Glynis, (we'd been close friends for 21 years) and I were e-mailing each other. I confided to her how frightened I was. She told me that she was praying for me. A few days later Glynis said that she was going to come out to be with me the weekend before my surgery up through the day after my surgery. I was so relieved that she was coming out. Maria loved her and I knew that she would feel safe with her.

On the Friday before my surgery I finally had my will notarized and had the funds transferred into the bank account to pay for my surgery's insurance co-pay. Glynis was coming into town later on that afternoon. Everything was going as planned. She came over on Saturday and we visited, laughed, cried and prayed together.

On Sunday, the day before my total thyroidectomy, Maria and I laughed and hugged throughout the day. I told her many times that day how much I loved her. I tried my best to hide from her how frightened I was to go under the knife. God really gave me peace that day before my surgery. The day was coming to an end. Before I went to sleep I prayed, *"Father God, please help me to sleep well tonight. Please go before me for tomorrow's surgery. Guide my surgeons' hands. Let it be a successful surgery. Please let me survive so that I can watch my daughter grow up. In Jesus name, Amen."*

As I sat in the utter darkness of despair the dazzling light of hope and life became brighter. The life that I was choosing would be different than what I was accustomed to but I wanted to choose life and live my life to the fullest. I decided that I would not let my fear of Graves' disease hold me in darkness any longer. I refused to let Graves' disease rob me of a life filled with my daughter's beauty and the beauty of a life chosen to live in wonder of each new day.

I invite you to continue with me on my journey of living with Graves' disease in my next book which begins in the early morning of the day of my total thyroidectomy. You will experience my memories of the first moments I woke up from surgery and the disappointments and joys of the miraculous outcome of my surgery.

BOOK

TWO

Emerging from the Cave
Surviving Graves' Disease

Emerging From the CAVE

Surviving Graves' Disease

CELIA MARIE

Celia Marie, LLC
2020

For Ri and my Papa

Ri: you are so amazing and your strength, optimism and courage
are an inspiration to me. You are the light of my life. I love you, Ri.
Papa: Richard Duron La Paglia, 1924-1979, you are my hero. I look
at the brightest star and know it's you smiling on me and encouraging
me each step of the way.

Acknowledgements

Katie Knapp edited my first book, Life in the Cave Overwhelming Graves' Disease, and I am forever grateful to her. She helped me to reach deeper and higher and was with me every step of the way as I strove to draw my readers into my thoughts and emotions during my experience of life in the cave.

Glynis Bonser has continued to be my special friend patiently listening, praying, crying and laughing with me on my journey of emerging from life in the cave. A friend loveth at all times. Proverbs 17:17

Deb Lowe has encouraged me since we were friends in second grade. She knows me better than most and continues to be a source of enthusiasm and joy! You have always been an inspiration to me, Deb.

Pat has provided the necessary medical insurance, paid for medical procedures, the doctor's visits, and prescriptions. Thank you.

Barb has rolled up her sleeves and not been afraid to help me during the most challenging of circumstances throughout our long friendship. I appreciate you, Barb.

My brother Pat was willing to come into the cave with me which helped me to not feel so alone in those early days. His visits in the beginning of this journey were my lifeline. The laughter we shared during the hours leading up to my surgery was exactly what I needed. Pat, you are the most amazing brother on the planet and I love you so much. Numbers 6:24-26 is one of my most favorite verses, too.

Eric has been a source of encouragement, strength and inspiration. Chase Cross. Gracias y bendiciones!

Introduction

You may have read my first book, Life in the Cave: Overcoming Grave's Disease, and have waited for months to learn of the details and outcome of my surgery. As promised, in this book I will begin with the first moments of the day of my surgery continuing my saga throughout the first year following my total thyroidectomy.

The two main reasons for choosing a total thyroidectomy are goiter (enlargement of the thyroid) and hyperthyroidism (overactive thyroid). In my case I had a huge goiter and severe hyperthyroidism. Two strikes against me. At one point my body was producing such an enormous amount of thyroxine that it could have kept fourteen people at a normal level. No wonder I couldn't relax, sit still, focus, and concentrate. My body was in a heightened state of activity all of the time. In addition to suffering from insomnia, I was a victim of nightmares, which caused an evening ritual of being perpetually wiped out, falling asleep and waking up in a total sweat from a panic attack. This cycle continued for over a year.

Due to the increasing size of my goiter, it began to press down on my windpipe, causing me to have difficulty breathing. My right lung was also affected and I was being treated for walking pneumonia. My skin was also becoming jaundiced as toxins flowed rampantly throughout my body. Sadly, I had the appearance of grave (no pun intended) illness because my vital organs were becoming poisoned. The combination of these medical issues presented a very serious challenge and it was the advanced stages of the goiter and hyperthyroidism that pointed to the only solution: a total thyroidectomy.

Although I did not want the total thyroidectomy I could no longer do the simplest of activities. Walking, standing, and sitting up and down were accomplished only with the greatest difficulty. In spite of these challenges, my surgeons were very optimistic that my body would tolerate the surgery well and heal properly. I had to trust their expertise and professional opinion. Their enthusiasm and confidence provided the glimmer of hope that I needed.

At this point I'd like to list the symptoms of Graves' disease. They include anxiety, brittle hair, fatigue, frequent bowel movements, goiter, increase in perspiration, insomnia, irritability, rapid/irregular heartbeat, sensitivity to heat, and weight loss. Further, Graves' Opthalmopathy and Graves' Dermopathy are two conditions that Graves' disease patients may experience. The symptoms of Graves' Opthalmopathy are excessive tearing (sensation of grit or sand in either/both eyes) reddened/inflamed eyes, widening of the space between eyelids, swelling of the lids and tissues around the eyes, and light sensitivity. My condition has definitely improved since my total thyroidectomy but I still experience the tearing, reddened eyes and light sensitivity. The symptoms of Graves' Dermopathy are reddening/swelling of the skin, often on shins and top of feet. It has been two years since my surgery and I have seen little improvement and healing of my shins and top of my feet. I will share with you my personal experiences with each of these symptoms. Every case is unique, though, and you or your loved one may not have each of these symptoms.

Looking back it was the spring of 2006 that finally yielded all of the above symptoms. The anxiety was noticeable to others by then. For example, my boss walked into my classroom and said, "Celia, you are anxious, aren't you?" In addition, I was fatigued to the point of falling asleep at work as Tiffany, my outgoing and cheerful student, would giggle shouting "teacher, wake up!", a coworker commented and teased me about my frequent trips to the bathroom, and two coworkers told me a few times that my neck area looked swollen.

Compliments on my much slimmer body began during the summer of 2005 and continued through the spring of 2006. Even though it was exciting to receive praise for the huge amount, nearly forty pounds, of weight loss it was a negative symptom because my body was in an acute hyperactive state of metabolism. My hair began falling out in March of 2006, too. I was also experiencing severe sensitivity to heat and, beginning as early as February, I wore shorts and short sleeve tops. The inability to sleep at night was becoming more frequent. Crankiness might as well have been my middle name, along with the continual rapid heartbeat which was alarming to me. All of these symptoms were an indication of Graves' disease and hyperthyroidism during September of 2006.

The purpose of writing my first book was to reach out to that one person who knew that something was dreadfully wrong with their body but was paralyzed with fear and chose not to seek medical attention. I wanted to share how the fear that gripped me made it much more difficult for my body to withstand and heal from this autoimmune disorder. My daughter, my husband, my family members and close friends, along with my coworkers, were all negatively affected by my decision to not seek early medical intervention. I know full well how fear can totally grip and paralyze you and I also know what it's like to see hurt, despair and fear affect those closest to you because you are stuck in a moment you can't find a way out of.

My main purpose in writing Emerging From the Cave is to share with you the joys and disappointments of the outcome of my total thyroidectomy and reveal how my life has continued to change in the past two years. I hope that medical professionals (doctors, nurses, phlebotomists, ultrasound technicians, nursing students, surgeons, endocrinologists and autoimmune disorder researchers) will find this book helpful in seeing the humanity of the Graves' disease patient and I pray that you, the Graves' disease patient or loved one, will find encouragement and hope within the pages of this book you are reading in your hands, or on your wireless device or perhaps even listening to via audio book as you drive.

Graves' disease is a treatable but not curable autoimmune disease. At the time of this writing there is still no cure for Graves' disease. I hope that I will be living when a cure is found. I do not wish this disease upon anyone because this is a life altering condition that affects all facets of your being. I believe that we all have four important components in our being: physical, mental, emotional and spiritual. Graves' disease affects each of these areas. I have found that when I nurture all of these areas I am surviving and overcoming Graves' disease.

If you have read Life in the Cave Overcoming Graves' Disease you will know that my spiritual being was what I tapped into when I had hit rock bottom with no place to go but up. Although this book will focus more on physical, mental and emotional areas I want to share with you that prayer and scripture reading continue to be a daily part of my life. I do believe in physical healing although I have not yet been fully healed of Graves' disease. If you believe in the power of prayer, please join me in praying that a cure for Graves' disease is found.

I want to publicly thank Dr. Richard Harding and Dr. Bryce, my amazing thyroidectomy surgeons and the beautiful nurse of color who gently, carefully took care of me during my first twelve hours after surgery and treated me with the utmost respect and dignity as my body came out of the anesthesia. I am so sorry that I do not remember your name but you are my hero. I hope that you will always be successful in your nursing career. I salute you.

I would also like to salute the small population (mostly women) who daily battle Graves' disease. A portion of the proceeds of this book goes to the National Graves' Disease and Thyroid Foundation located in Rancho Santa Fe, California. It is my deepest desire that you will receive information that will challenge you to learn even more about Graves' disease and join us in achieving Graves' disease awareness in our homes, communities, states and the world.

Celia Marie
May 2010

Chapter One
February 25, 2008

It was a beautiful morning and the sun shone brightly. The air was slightly chilly, yet pleasant. I lay peacefully in bed for a moment before I remembered that this was the day I was to go in for my total thyroidectomy. I immediately began to fight waves of panic as my mind began racing with the thought of what if I die during surgery? I attempted to calm myself down with positive thoughts and thankfulness that I had two experienced surgeons whom I trusted performing my surgery. Now that I was calm I leaned over to say good morning to our Australian Cattle Dog, Boomer, who was lying peacefully on his very own leather bed right beside me.

I walked into Ri's bedroom and gently woke up my daughter, gave her a kiss and told her that I loved her. I reminded her that today was my surgery and we needed to get ready to go to the hospital. Glynis (my longtime friend of twenty-one years) was driving over to meet us and would follow us to the hospital. I had packed my overnight bag the night before and included my CD player along with my Best of Sixpence None the Richer CD. We put my belongings in the car and waited for Glynis to arrive. While we were waiting, I said goodbye to Boomer, Jade (my lynx point Siamese cat) and Snickers (my daughter's bunny rabbit). Tears were in my eyes and a huge lump was in my throat as I hugged each of them. They were more than pets—they were family.

Glynis drove up right on time and after we greeted each other with hugs, exchanged a little bit of small talk and then decided which route was best to take, we all got into our separate cars and drove to Banner Thunderbird hospital in Glendale, AZ. We went to the admitting area and waited about ten minutes before I met with a hospital staff person who asked me to provide personal information along with a copy of my will. I signed several documents and paid hundreds of dollars for my hospital stay co-pay. It seems like it took around twenty minutes for the complete admitting process and then we walked to the waiting room area. I was surprised that the nurse called me in to the pre-op room within less than five minutes after arriving.

Much to my disappointment, no one was allowed to come in with me while I waited as they prepared the room for me. I sat in a chair for at least fifteen minutes before the nurse actually called me into my pre-op room. I was instructed to undress and put on a hospital gown as the medical assistant closed the curtain.

Several minutes later my nurse asked me, through the closed curtain, if I needed any help and I replied "yes, I do." She opened the curtain and when I turned around I realized that she was Emily, the mom of one of my students. I was surprised and delighted to discover that Emily was going to be my nurse. It is such a small world.

As Emily and I chatted about Claire I began to relax. I asked to see a picture of Claire and Emily obliged. It had been two years since I had seen Claire or Emily. While Emily wrote down my vitals I looked at the walls of my room. It was decorated in a beach theme. I was so humbled that God even orchestrated the smallest of things to make me comfortable. During college I loved surfing; in fact, my bedroom was decorated with a surfer's beach theme. I was extremely thankful to God for arranging the beach-themed hospital room for me because it was familiar, comforting and helped me to relax.

After I settled in, Ri and Glynis came to visit me. About an hour later my brother, Pat, stopped by. We talked and laughed a lot. We had always gotten along well together and this day was no different. After he left Ri and Glynis came back to sit with me again. My surgery was scheduled for 1:00 pm but around 12:30 pm a new nurse (Emily's shift had recently ended) informed me that Dr. Harding and Dr. Bryce were running behind schedule.

An x-ray was ordered for my right lung because I was having breathing complications. After the x-ray was performed we waited and waited for the results. Ri and Glynis decided to get lunch at the hospital cafeteria and while they were eating my brother came back in to see me. The results of the lung x-ray were not good. Dr. Harding wanted to postpone the surgery for a few more hours to see if my lung would improve.

Truthfully, I was hoping that Dr. Harding would decide I was too ill and weak to perform the surgery. We waited until around 3:00 pm before another x-ray of my lung was taken. Two hours later Dr. Harding came in to discuss the results with me. He said that my lung was marginally better but because my goiter was huge it was causing my trachea area to collapse which explained why I was having extreme difficulty breathing along with the complications of my right lung. My skin also appeared jaundiced. Dr. Harding said that if he didn't perform the surgery that day he was uncertain if I would pull through because I was critically ill. He decided that he and Dr. Bryce would perform my total thyroidectomy at 6:00 pm. My surgery would be their last surgery of the day.

A few minutes before my surgery, Pat (Ri's dad) came in to see me for about five minutes. After he left, Ri and Glynis stayed with me until the nurse placed the anesthesia in my I.V. Within approximately five minutes after administering the anesthesia, the nurse wheeled me out of my pre-op room as I waved goodbye to Ri and Glynis, telling Ri that I loved her.

Chapter Two
February 26, 2008

After telling Ri that I loved her as the nurse was wheeling me out of my pre-op room, my next thought was that I must have survived the surgery because I was awake. (Actually, nine hours had passed since I had fallen asleep). Praise God, I'm going to see Ri grow up after all! I was so thankful to God for allowing me to survive the surgery as tears welled up in my eyes. I looked at the clock and it was around 3:00 am.

Huge waves of nausea overtook me while I was looking at the clock and I began to vomit everywhere. I was so humiliated and embarrassed. I tried to apologize to the nurse but could barely speak. I didn't realize yet that a hose was crammed down deep into my throat and trachea area. I continued to vomit and began to cry because I felt ashamed about being violently ill in front of the nurse. She assured me that there was no need to apologize. I fell asleep after that.

When I woke up I was staring at a hole in the wall. All of the meds I was taking made me feel groggy, nauseated, and like I was in a fog. I couldn't even speak above a whisper. I slowly realized that I was hooked up to several monitors along with oxygen tubes in my nostrils. It was very uncomfortable to be limited in mobility because of all of the various tubes and hoses connected to my body and a myriad of machines. I fell asleep again. Someone woke me up to tell me that they needed to take an x-ray of my right lung. I tried to move as best as I could but I was weak and miserable. I then fell back asleep.

The next time I woke up Ri and Pat were coming into my ICU room. Ri looked terribly frightened to see all of the hoses and tubes connected to me. My eyes were still bulging and I had a huge gauze bandage covering my neck area; two drains had also been placed in my neck where the goiter had been removed. I truly believed that I must have looked like an alien. Later, Pat told me that I looked dreadful; even the nurses seemed appalled at my appearance but these ICU nurses were always kind, gentle and respectful towards me. Pat described my appearance as a holocaust survivor which meant that even though I was technically alive, I looked dead.

I was overjoyed to see Ri but equally sobered and concerned to see her frightened expression at my appearance. She slowly walked over to me and offered me a beautiful, soft, white polar bear that I could hold on to for comfort. Ri is exceptionally sweet and thoughtful. I was extremely proud of my kind and loving daughter. She also brought me a get well card with a picture of a puppy with a band-aid on his forehead. The card was "signed" by all of our pets along with Ri and Pat. I smiled and tried to laugh as I read the card. I still have that card on my dresser as a reminder of the love that surrounded me the morning after my surgery and still does.

I drifted in and out of sleep. I asked Ri if we were waiting for me to go in for my surgery and she replied, "No, Mom, they did your surgery yesterday." I was understandably confused from all of the meds they were giving me and also drained from the physical trauma that my body underwent during my total thyroidectomy.

After the next round of meds, Glynis came to see me for a few minutes before she drove back to California. I was sad to see her leave because I appreciated her for taking time out of her busy schedule to be with Ri during my surgery and I also enjoyed her company. We have always found something to laugh about even in the most stressful situations. This hospital scenario was no different.

About an hour after Glynis left, my brother Pat came to see me. He looked awfully concerned when he saw me for the first time after my surgery. It was quite humiliating to have my loved ones see me looking horrible but I was exceedingly thankful that they were there with me. I couldn't speak to them very well because my vocal chords were very sore from the surgery and the trachea tube was jabbed down my throat. I appreciated seeing their faces with their love shining in their eyes for me.

I drifted in and out of sleep for the rest of the day. Ri and Pat came back to visit me during the evening hours. I discovered that there were even IVs in my feet and I was also hooked up to a catheter. All of this was so humiliating to me. My ICU nurse was extremely kind and respectful towards me. She made sure to keep me cleaned up (I was still vomiting a lot). She smelled so nice. I was exceedingly blessed to have her as my nurse during the first day after surgery and I sadly whispered goodbye when her shift ended.

After meeting my evening nurse I quickly discovered that she was very efficient and kind as she asked me what she could do to make me comfortable. Earlier in the day I had decided that I no longer wanted to be in ICU and requested to be moved to a private room several times during the day but my surgeons and pulmonary doctor didn't believe that I was strong enough. Being the tenacious person that I am, I asked my new nurse if I could be moved to a private room and she told me that she would find out. My vitals were taken and after about an hour and a half she came back and said that a private room was being prepared for me. I was relieved and thankful. She removed my catheter and helped me into the restroom.

While I was in the restroom a thin pinkish bloody fluid began leaking from the huge gauze bandage in my neck area. I was alarmed as I pushed the emergency button for the nurse. She helped me get all cleaned up. Once again I was humiliated to be in this offensive condition. I apologized to her (although it was very difficult for me to speak) for the mess and she graciously said that no apology was necessary. She then helped me get seated in the chair because I didn't want to lie down in the bed as I waited for the wheelchair to be delivered to my ICU room in order to be transported to my private room.

Around 10 pm I rode in the wheelchair to my new room. My nurse was in her early 20s and she commented on my daughter's Christy Miller book that was placed on the nightstand. She went on to say that she liked the music I was playing. I told her that the band was Sixpence None the Richer and she commented that she had heard of them and liked them. She then asked me if I wanted morphine for the pain and I hastily and emphatically replied "no." I was scared to take morphine because I saw how it had negatively affected Carole, my mother-in-law, when she was administered it during her last stage of lung cancer.

At 10:30 pm I asked the young nurse if Ri could spend the night with me and she said that Ri was not old enough to stay. I was extremely disappointed as I hugged Ri goodnight telling her I loved her. Ri and I have always been close and I didn't want to spend the night by myself in my private room. I was scared that something could go wrong and I wanted Ri with me as much as possible. I waved goodnight to her and we signed "I love you" to each other as she walked out of the hospital room. I then cried and looked at her Christy Miller book on my nightstand while I listened to Leigh Bingham Nash's soothing voice sing "Trust in the Lord' along with the brilliant talents of the Sixpence None the Richer musicians in the background.

When my nurse came in to check on me I asked her if she would help me as I tried to prop my neck area/head on the bed because there was no way that I could lie flat. It was very difficult to get in and out of the hospital bed and my incision area continued to ooze the thin pinkish body fluid. My nurse gave me a new hospital gown because the fluid kept leaking onto my gown. After I finally got settled in my new room I tried to go to sleep. Impossible. I didn't like to be alone and I was still in pain from the surgery feeling horrible and blurry from all of the meds that I was taking.

Chapter Three
February 27, 2008

I finally dozed off and was awakened by someone wanting to take another x-ray of my lung. Once again it took me awhile to drift off to sleep and then another young nurse came in to take my vitals. Lovely. It was now 3:00 am and I didn't want to be in the hospital anymore. I missed Ri, Boomer, Snickers and Jade. I couldn't sleep. It was just too noisy in the hospital.

Around 6:00 am Dr Bryce (one of my surgeons) came in to see how I was doing. He had also checked on me while I was in ICU. He talked to me for quite a while and told me that I had given him and Dr. Harding (my primary surgeon) a run for their money as my surgery was the second liveliest/bloodiest that Dr. Harding had ever performed but they were up for it and I was up for it. He went on to say that they were able to remove all of the goiter and it was about three times the size of a healthy thyroid—no wonder I was ill and having such difficulty breathing.

Dr. Bryce then proceeded to remove the drains from my neck and I almost passed out when I saw how long the tubes were that had been inside my neck. His next step was to put a clean gauze bandage over my incision. He told me to wash the area with antibacterial soap daily. At the time I had no idea how hideous I still looked and now I have the utmost respect for him because he treated me with a great amount of respect and concern while sitting on the edge of my hospital bed just hours after my surgery. You see, my eyes were terribly swollen, red and watery. My face was very puffy. I had a huge bandage over my neck area which concealed a fresh three and a half inch incision that was oozing a thin, pinkish liquid. Within this incision area the surgeons inserted two drains. I had repeatedly vomited after my total thyroidectomy and hadn't been able to brush my teeth. I also hadn't been given the opportunity to have my hair brushed. Although I'm certain I looked exceedingly ugly, we chatted (I mostly listened because I could only speak in a whisper) for a few minutes more before he told me that he would come back and check on me. After Dr. Bryce left, my pulmonary specialist came in to see how I was doing. He informed me that he had been monitoring my lungs hours before my surgery (especially the right one) and that during surgery the right lung had completely shut down. He went on to say that he was going to continue to monitor it throughout the day. About an hour after he left, Ri and Pat came to visit. Pat stayed for a few minutes and then informed me that he was going to show properties (he's a realtor) to one of his clients. Ri stayed with me all day and I was thankful to have her with me. Ri asked me if I needed anything as she held my hand. She is such a joy to be with and I enjoy her cheerful and easygoing personality. She was going to be twelve years old within a few weeks time and I was very proud of the way that she was handling my surgery and hospital stay.

I was also thankful that my friend Glynis came out from San Diego to be with Ri during my surgery. I asked Glynis to share her perspective on the waiting room along with the next morning after my surgery and this is what she had to say:

"Ri and I waved goodbye to Celia as she was rolled out of the prep room and taken to the operating room. I breathed another prayer for her, but in my heart knew that was going to come through this. As we walked down the hall I put my arm around Maria's shoulders and gave her a little hug.

In the waiting room Ri was kept occupied with the few toys she had brought with her, but the pillow and the blanket are what gave her comfort. She and her dad Pat took a few walks outside of the room and I bought her some candy out of the machine that was conveniently located nearby.

Celia's brother Pat was there and the two of us had some serious dialogue about his baby sister. As I saw the concern in his eyes and heard the worry in his voice, it dawned on me how much he truly loved and cared for Celia Marie. It touched my heart.

As the time marched on I kept praying for Celia, and the men kept checking to see if the surgeons were going to come out and talk to us soon. Finally, someone came and got us and took us to an area just outside the double swinging doors where the doctors would emerge and give us the news about Celia.

The surgeons came out and we anxiously listened to every word. Celia was in recovery and doing fine! Dr. Harding smiled victoriously and chuckled in disbelief when he told us that Celia's was the bloodiest thyroid surgery he had ever done and that he had been doing this for thirteen years. He told us that the goiter was huge and a bleeder. I prayed within myself thanking our loving Heavenly Father for the success of the surgery and petitioning Him for Celia's recovery.

With lighter hearts we headed to the parking lot. Ri and her dad separated from Pat and me as we continued to go towards our cars. Pat was so relieved that his sister was doing okay and was telling me how special and beautiful Celia was.

The next morning I came by to see Celia before I headed back home to San Diego. I walked into her ICU room and there she lay weak, sick and miserable with tubes and machines all around her. My heart went out to her. She looked like she hurt on every inch of her body. Her neck was so bandaged up that it looked as if she couldn't move it. Her eyes were swollen and watery and it was all she could do to get out a whisper. I could tell that it hurt her to talk. Celia's husband and daughter were there with her so I didn't stay long. I knew she needed to rest so I prayed with her and assured her that although she had a long road ahead of her, she was going to be okay and would get better." Thank you, Glynis, for sharing your perspective with us.

Around 11:00 am I desperately wanted to leave the hospital and I asked the nurse if I could be discharged. She came back to say, "No, your levels aren't stable enough to be released." I was very disappointed. A few hours later I again asked if I could leave. She said that she would contact my surgeons to see if it could be arranged. My levels had finally improved enough and they agreed to release me on the condition that I would faithfully take calcium pills because my calcium level was borderline. I promised that I would.

I asked if I could take a shower and the nurse brought me shampoo, soap, a towel and washcloth. It was one of the most challenging showers that I have ever taken in my life because I had to be very careful around the incision area. I was still very weak. Once I finished my shower and got dressed I looked in the mirror. I looked repulsive. My eyes were still bulging. My face was very puffy and red. The gauze over my neck area looked awful. I started to cry. I thought that my appearance would improve once I had the surgery. In actually, I looked worse than I did before the surgery. I was extremely disappointed and so very tired of being ugly.

Around 3:00 pm I was relieved when the nurse brought my discharge papers for me to sign. In less than a half-hour I was in the car and heading home. It was a record-breaking heat day in the 90s and it was very hot in the car. I didn't care, though, because I was out of that noisy hospital.

Chapter Four
Home at Last

I slowly and carefully got out of the car with Maria's help and walked to the door. I don't remember who unlocked the door but I saw Boomer through the glass windows of the French door waiting on the other side. When I opened the door he greeted me with a friendly bark then he started whimpering and I started crying while I attempted to hug him. We were locked in this moment of time completely unaware of anything else but each other. I realized then how much Boomer loved me and how much I loved him. From that moment on, Boomer has been my greatest protector and companion. Ri and Pat said that he continually looked for me all throughout the house during my hospital stay. I never realized the special bond that Boomer and I had formed until we were separated. Boomer is my forever friend. I was so thankful to be reunited with him and grateful to be home.

I walked slowly into the kitchen with Boomer by my side. He wanted to be right beside me and that comforted me. It seemed so surreal to be at home. I was still pumped up with all of the meds given to me at the hospital and I felt like I was having some out-of-body experience as I looked around like I was seeing all of my familiar surroundings for the first time through another person's eyes.

As I walked down the hallway to my bedroom my eyes welled up with tears. The best way I can describe what I was feeling is to compare it with the way a runner may feel when participating in a very challenging marathon. The runner is halfway through the marathon and doesn't want to turn back now but is weary and knows he's only halfway there. I had hoped to come home with normal looking eyes, a thinner face, healthy looking hair and a slimmer body. Instead I was in physical pain from the incision, along with emotional pain from my unrealistic expectations. I was angry that my life wasn't going to ever be the way it was before this ominous autoimmune disease attacked my body.

Now that I was in my bedroom I tried to get into bed but it was such a challenging task. I had propped up several pillows to elevate my head because there was no way that I could lay down flat. The incision in my neck area was larger than my surgeons anticipated and they explained that they had to cut further into my muscle tissue due to the size of the goiter. As a result, the muscles in my neck and shoulder area were very sore. I could barely move my neck sided to side without experiencing a great deal of pain. I finally got settled in and fell asleep for a few hours. I woke up and slowly walked to the family room while Boomer followed closely behind me. I sat in the oversized leather chair and wished that the physical pain in my neck area would just go away. It didn't. I started having that bizarre out-of-body sensation all over again but because the pain was so intense I found myself compelled to take another pain pill. Throughout the night I slept, woke up, dozed, got up to take some more meds and then fell back into a troubled sleep.

I don't remember what time I woke up the next morning. But I do know that even though my first full day home from the hospital was a blur it was good to be home. I saw Snickers for the first time and he seemed happy to see me, too. I smiled as I reached down to pet him. I was immediately overwhelmed with intense pain. It hurt to bend down. I still hadn't seen Jade and was eager to talk to her and pet her soft fur.

Throughout the day Ri asked me if I needed anything. She was a great help to me with whatever task I was unable to do. After I drifted in and out of sleep during the day, I needed to change my gauze dressing. That proved to be a daunting task as I tried to put the sterile gauze square on top of the incision then attempted to cut the tape to secure the gauze dressing with only one hand while the other held up the sterile gauze square. Frustrating.

The day consisted of taking meds at assigned times and trying to eat. My trachea area was incredibly sore from the trachea tube. Eating pudding was painful and drinking liquid was too. The calcium pills that I had been prescribed were huge and it hurt to swallow them. The effects that the trachea tube had left on my throat and windpipe area irritated me. I didn't like the nausea I was experiencing. I had to remind myself to be grateful that the surgery was behind me and better days were ahead of me.

It continued to be a challenge to get in and out of bed but I still slept a lot. At bedtime I decided to try to sleep in the oversized leather chair in the family room. Boomer joined me by sleeping on the leather love seat beside me. After waking up several times that night I slowly walked back to the bedroom and propped up the pillows and got into bed. I awoke about an hour later with a severe panic attack. I decided right then and there to stop taking the pain pill. I hated having panic attacks. I still felt like an alien and was tired of having the out-of-body sensation feelings. I never took a pain pill after that night.

Chapter Five
Hypothyroidism

The first week home proved to be more challenging than I had anticipated. As I gazed at my reflection in the mirror after I had taken my shower I gasped at the huge bruises on my chest area, my shoulders and my upper arms. I looked like I was pummeled badly in a street fight and I had lost. I wondered if perhaps I had flat-lined during surgery.

I was irritated that I was not getting stronger by now and I could barely talk above a whisper. It literally hurt to try to project my voice. I could not talk loud enough to have a conversation on the phone and I was still too weak to get on the internet to read e-mails and go on MySpace to communicate with family and friends. Totally frustrating.

Finally, on the fourth day after my surgery, I was strong enough to check my e-mails. I had received hundreds and I found it to be too daunting to read through them all. I scanned through them and answered the ones from family and close friends. I also tried to talk on the phone but could only talk for a couple of minutes because it hurt my vocal chords to speak. At least I could communicate through e-mail and MySpace so that was encouraging.

On Tuesday at 9:00 am I met with Dr. Harding for my complimentary post-op consultation. Dr. Harding was optimistic, enthusiastic and encouraging as he talked to me while examining my neck area. He asked me to repeat vowel sounds after him and observed that I was having difficulty sounding out the vowels. Although I was concerned about this struggle he reassured me that my vocal chords were healing and I would, in time, master the correct pronunciation of the vowels.

Dr. Harding went on to share with me the test results were in and said the words I had been praying to hear since

2006: "Celia, there was not a bit of cancer in your goiter". He went on to say "and we meticulously removed and scraped the entire goiter out." Tears welled up in my eyes as I exclaimed, "Praise God, thank you Dr. Harding!" I saw the joy in his eyes and the sense of accomplishment on his face that he was satisfied with a job well done. As I quickly looked over at Ri to see her response to the good news she looked relieved, excited and had a tear in her eye as it dawned on her that her mother was not going to die from thyroid cancer.

Our drive home was filled with shouts of "awesome" and "thank you, Jesus" in the car as we travelled from downtown Phoenix back to Glendale. I don't think I ever stopped praising God all the way home. For two years I had been paralyzed with fear that I had thyroid cancer and to have that burden which weighed a million tons lifted off of me was totally phenomenal. I wish I could articulate exactly what this freedom from the fear of cancer meant to me. The chains from the mental and emotional oppression and torment were released and the shackles from the paralysis of fear were broken off of my being. It also brought me great joy to see the change of countenance in Ri. She lifted her face upward, squared her shoulders back in confidence and walked with a lighter step. The good news that I had not a bit of cancer was also a testimony of the power of prayer and faith to Ri and me.

I reflected back to my meetings with Dr. Duick (my second endocrinologist) and Dr. Harding and they both concurred that without a thyroid my body would go hypothyroid. I was praying that the Lord would spare me and heal my body from having to experience hypothyroidism. He had other plans for me, though.

I wasn't looking forward to the eleven symptoms of hypothyroidism which are brittle hair, depression, dry skin, elevated blood cholesterol level, fatigue, increased sensitivity to cold, muscle aches, tenderness, stiffness, muscle weakness, puffy face, sluggishness, and weight gain.

I did not experience the above symptoms the minute my thyroid was removed. Over time, though, I began to have symptoms of hypothyroidsm and now, two years later, I have all of the hypothyroidism symptoms. Muscle aches, tenderness, stiffness and weakness occurred almost immediately following the surgery.

The muscle aches were to the level of pain that I would cry out in misery. I would cry because my muscles would cramp up so bad. The pain was unbearable and I could not move the muscle involved. This could occur in any muscle at any time. The most prevalent area, though, was the back of my legs, my feet and my toes. I would also experience horrific muscle cramps in my chest cavity area and the back of my neck. I never knew when the muscle cramps were going to start and I had no way to prepare for them. Sometimes they would strike at the grocery store, at home, at the movies or at church. It was frightening when they would suddenly come upon me in the shower. I had to constantly take extra precautions in the shower for fear that I would fall and strike my head during the fall.

Sluggishness was another symptom I faced immediately after my surgery. I kept complaining to my endocrinologist about the sluggishness and he finally prescribed Cytomel in July of 2008. Two years later I am still taking Cytomel daily. Cytomel is a synthetic form of a natural thyroid hormone. I am now hypothyroid because I no longer have a thyroid and the Synthroid (thyroid hormone drug) isn't producing enough of the thyroid hormone that my body needs to function. Most patients who undergo a thyroidectomy will wind up being hypothyroid after their thyroid has been surgically removed.

Many months following the total thyroidectomy I noticed my hair beginning to grow back and although I was elated to have hair again I was disappointed that my hair was growing back thin and brittle. My hair used to be thick and wavy. To this day my hair is thin and brittle. It is just another reality that I've had to accept while surviving Graves' disease. While my hair was falling out I would wear fashionable hats. It was fun going to the department stores to try on hats. I still have the hats and they are a reminder of how far I've come.

In 2009 I began a naturopathic approach to dealing with elevated cholesterol levels and increased insulin levels. I began cardio and strength training which consisted of an urban belly dance workout and a George Foreman regimen. I stopped drinking caffeinated beverages and eliminated soda. I started eating more servings of fresh, steamed veggies and added freshly squeezed lemon to my water. My goal was to drink 64 ounces of water daily. I still incorporate all of these natural remedies in my daily activities. Unfortunately in February of 2010, despite the naturopathic therapy, my cholesterol and insulin levels were still too high so my doctor prescribed Crestor (synthetic lip-lowering agent) and Metformin (antihyperglycemic agent). It is now June of 2010 and I am still taking these meds daily in addition to the naturopathic regiment which also consists of aromatherapy.

Dry skin has been a huge issue for me, especially in my lower legs and feet. I have never had the most attractive feet and it has been embarrassing to have them look even worse with the acute dry skin problem. I use Eucerin Dry Skin Therapy Everyday Protection Body Lotion with SPF15 and this product is very effective in moisturizing and protecting my skin.

My face and neck area continues to be combination (normal/oily) along with myxedema prominent on both my left and right cheeks which causes redness. I have found that Clinique Dramatically Different Moisturizing Lotion has worked wonders on my facial skin. I have not found a remedy for my puffy face, though, much to my chagrin.

I noticed the increased sensitivity to cold during 2009. When I was hyperthyroid I would wear shorts and sleeveless tops in the winter but now I wear sweaters and jeans while everyone else is sporting shorts and sleeveless tops!

Because I already battled depression with the Graves' disease and hyperthyroidism I don't believe that going hypothyroid impacted me that much. Whenever I would feel the depression coming on I would remind myself how much I really believe that laughter is one of the best ways to combat depression. I enjoy comedies and humorous books. I also enjoy laughing with Ri and my close friends Glynis and Barb.

When I was in college one of my psychology professors shared that he conducted a study on humor therapy and the results of his study revealed that humor is conducive to evoking a happier and more positive sense of wellbeing. If you are struggling with depression I highly recommend that you read humorous books, watch comedies, listen to upbeat music and look at the cup half full as often as possible. An attitude of gratitude is very important. Make a list of everything that you are thankful for and refer to your list daily. Positive thoughts are more powerful than negativity. A thankful heart is a happy heart. Laughter, smiles and positive thoughts produce endorphins which uplift your mood.

Weight gain hasn't affected me much since I have become hypothyroid. What I deal with now is metabolism issues. Because my insulin production is way off my metabolism is practically non-existent. No matter how much I workout and reduce calories I am unable to lose weight. This metabolism malady is my Waterloo. I have shared my concerns with my doctor and he stated that the Metformin should help jump-start my metabolism. It's been two months since I've been on Metformin and I've yet to see even one ounce of weight loss.

Each of us is different and if you've been diagnosed with hypothyroidism you may not have all of the symptoms I've listed and discussed. In most situations these symptoms can be effectively treated. I feel compelled to point out that only you truly know your body and if you are unhappy with the results of the medication your doctor has prescribed for you make sure you speak up. It doesn't matter what the test results indicate. If you're not feeling right you may need to get your dosage adjusted. You may even have to find another doctor who will listen to your concerns. Look out for yourself because you're the only one who knows exactly how you are doing.

Chapter Six
Social Security Disability Process

You may be experiencing severe stress because of a lack of income. A possible income solution available to you if you are unable to work is social security disability. There are three stages of the social security disability process. They are application, decision, and appeals process. Two optional and additional steps are retaining legal counsel and the appeals decision. This was indeed one of the most stressful and grievous issues of my battle with Graves' disease and hyperthyroidism.

I turned in my resignation on June 9, 2006 and was too fatigued to even look for a part-time job. It was now November of 2006 and we were beginning to feel the financial crunch of being a one income family. During a phone conversation my friend Barb suggested that I consider filing for social security disability. I thanked her for the suggestion and told her that I would think about it. I really didn't want to go this route but I was in such bad, physical shape that this looked like my only option.

I went online to discover how to start the whole social security disability process. Please keep in mind that I was in an acute state of confusion and lack of focus was an everyday occurrence. It took everything I had to read the instructions on how to apply for disability. It literally took hours for me to comprehend what I was supposed to do. I had to take frequent breaks because my eyes teared up often as I attempted to read the words on the computer screen. Finally, on November 5, 2006, with much trepidation, I was ready to begin filing for social security disability. I applied online. They demanded a plethora of information, job history, medical history and a myriad of other information to complete the online application. Eight hours later I was finished but the utter frustration of the process left me in tears and total exhaustion.

The next step was to find out if the social security administration received my online application. I received an e-mail that it was indeed received. Great, I thought. I prayed that it would not take long to receive my social security disability payments. I didn't think much about it during the holidays because I was busy with the Radioactive Iodine (RAI) therapy on November 29, 2006, focusing on the holidays season and anticipating a positive outcome, dreaming of no more bulging eyes, no more rapid heartbeat, no more anxiety, no more insomnia and returning to my normal self.

Within two weeks of filing, I received a big manila envelope from social security instructing me to fill out the enclosed paperwork which needed to be sent to each doctor and medical provider who was involved in my case. It took several hours to complete the paperwork as it required that I list each provider involved and look up their mailing address, phone number, and give detailed information of the service that each provided. In mid-January I e-mailed Pam, my social security contact, and she confirmed that my file was being looked at but would take a few more weeks before a decision was made.

It was now March of 2007 but I received no news of a decision about my case. Nine months of being a single income family was definitely taking its toll. Thankfully we did not have car payments to make but we had real estate broker's fees that needed to be paid along with all of the realtor fees due (national, state, MLS, and Supra realtor fees). It upset me that we had to have a more toned-down birthday party for my daughter (her birthday is March 13) but she didn't complain.

The months went by and in May of 2007 I spoke to a Social Security Administration worker who informed me that he needed documentation from one of my doctors who had never responded to my original request for a doctor's report. I asked if this would have a negative effect on my case and he stated that it was almost the cut-off date for a decision to be made and he needed the documentation immediately.

My brother, Dan, e-mailed me frequently and asked how my social security application was coming along. As I shared with him my frustrations he responded that he and Pamelia (his wife) would continue to pray for me. He encouraged me to keep trusting the Lord.

Finally, during the month of June, I received the much-anticipated letter from social security. I anxiously opened the letter looking forward to a positive response. I was utterly disappointed to read that my request had been denied. The letter revealed that I could appeal the decision and gave instructions on how to begin the appeals process. I had no other choice but to appeal because I was still too ill to go back to work.

I filed the appeals paperwork and waited for direction on what to do next. I learned that the social security disability department was behind on their caseload and I had a feeling that I was going to be waiting a while for a response from them. In February of 2008 Pat began pressuring me to find out what was going on with my appeals so I called and spoke with the woman handling my case. She confirmed that they were still behind on their caseload. I shared the news with Pat and he became furious and began to shout at me that I wasn't doing enough and that I wasn't really sick, I was faking it because I just didn't want to work. Needless to say I was angry and hurt at his accusations. By this time I was totally fed up.

In May of 2008 I decided to contact the Caldwell and Ober law firm because their main focus was social security disability. Mark Caldwell agreed to take my case. I gave a plethora of information which included names, addresses, and phone numbers of endocrinologists, primary care physician, surgeons, ultra sound, thyroid scan uptake, x-ray technician, phlebotomist personnel along with the hospital information where both my Radioactive Iodine (RAI) therapy and total thyroidectomy were performed. Mr. Caldwell also needed dates of all of the services rendered along with a list of medications and dates they had been prescribed. It was truly like having a job preparing all of this information. Finally all of the paperwork was filed and now we waited for a date to meet with an administrative law judge.

During this period of waiting, I received phone calls from Dan and he would often pray with me during our phone conversations. The prayers helped to keep the flicker of light from emerging from the cave in my vision as I remained hopeful that there would be light at the end of the tunnel. My brother, Pat, continued to come by to visit me and we would often reminisce about our times together growing up which always included laughter and fond memories of our parents and siblings.

Meanwhile, we continued to struggle financially trying to just keep up with our basic monthly living expenses. The financial stress was unbearable and we continually fought over the lack of finances. I hated to see the negative effect all of the stress and fighting had on my daughter Maria. Pat demanded that I e-mail Congressman Trent Franks to tell him of my plight. I received a phone call and a letter from the Honorable Trent Franks office assuring me that they had contacted social security disability on my behalf. Within days I received a letter from social security disability stating they were behind but would be looking at my appeals case within the next few months.

The one flicker of hope was that with Mr. Caldwell representing me my appeals had a better chance of being found favorable by the administrative law judge. This helped me to calm down as I waited for my appeals hearing.

Six months later, on December 10, 2008 my daughter and I drove (my Saab 9 3 Convertible was smoking from under the hood and I had to stop the car and pull over to a safe place to fill the coolant twice because it was leaking) to the Social Security Administration building. My hearing was scheduled for 9:15 am. Two years and 1 month after I initially filed for social security disability benefits I finally met with an administrative law judge, along with my attorney Mark Caldwell.

If you have filed for social security disability benefits and you have been waiting years for a favorable decision, I strongly encourage you to consider retaining legal counsel. Do not give up. I know that it is stressful to fill out all of the paperwork that is required. It took me several hours every time I had to complete the required paperwork. Sometimes I would literally cry out of frustration while filling out the forms because it was hard to remember the information that was requested. I also struggled with lack of focus (I still do) while attempting to prepare the paperwork. It was very difficult for me to pursue the disability benefits but it was necessary due to the intense financial strain we were experiencing. My husband was working full-time as a cashier as well as working long hours as a licensed realtor. Additionally, the financial pressure was putting a huge strain on our marriage.

I am thankful that I met with my attorney before the hearing. He counseled me and helped me prepare. My actual hearing lasted less than a half hour. After the hearing, Mark Caldwell and I met to review. He informed me that it would be weeks before we would hear the administrative law judge's decision.

As Ri and I walked into the elevator I began to cry. The pressure of having to wait so long for this day was finally gone. Ri and I hugged each other and prayed that God would grant us favor with the administrative law judge. On the way out of the building my daughter and I stopped to admire the beautifully decorated Christmas tree on the main floor. Now we could officially celebrate the Christmas holiday!

It was now January 10, 2009, a month after my appeals hearing and I began looking for the letter from the administrative law judge in hopes of a favorable reply. Days before my birthday, as I opened the mailbox and scanned quickly through the letters, I spotted a thick envelope with Social Security Administration typed in the return address portion of the envelope. I walked into the house, told Ri the letter was here and we went into the kitchen and sat down at the kitchen table. I quickly opened the letter and began to scan the contents. My eyes were drawn to the decision that I had been waiting for since November 5, 2006. Unfavorable.

I was extremely disappointed. I had no idea how we were going to go on financially. We had exhausted all of our financial resources and the commission money from the real estate sales had long been gone and used to pay our basic living expenses. I dreaded telling Pat that my appeal was denied. I had figured that with all of the back disability payments I would be getting a lump sum of approximately $18,000 from social security. I was also angry because I had always worked, ever since I was eighteen years old, and we desperately needed the money. I wasn't trying to pull a scam on the government. I was only trying to financially provide for my twelve-year old daughter and alleviate some of the financial pressure from her father's shoulders.

Although the judge's ruling was a huge disappointment, to be truthful, I was relieved. Deep down I didn't want the label of being disabled. I wanted to return to my normal, healthy self. I wanted to be a positive contributor in the workforce. I wanted to use my God-given abilities and talents in a career. I didn't want this incurable disease to eliminate me from being gainfully employed.

I chose to trust God with this mountain of financial pressure. I chose to praise Him while I waited for an answer to our financial dilemma. I chose to take this setback and use it as a stepping stone as I continued to emerge from the cave.

Chapter Seven
Financial Pressures

My last day of full time work was June 9, 2006. We didn't have savings built up. Fortunately, Pat's employer, as a perk, paid our family medical insurance premiums. We were responsible for the doctors' visits, medical procedures and prescriptions co-pays, though. Additionally, an annual deductible must be met before we could take advantage of the percentage co-pays such as the hospital stay and actual total thyroidectomy.

Living on one income proved to be very challenging. The financial pressures became a point of contention with us. He resented the fact that I wasn't working and would regularly tell me that I was just faking it and that I wasn't sick. Further, I was just using it as an excuse to not work. These accusations deeply hurt me which caused problems to arise in other areas of our relationship. I would avoid him as much as possible because I abhorred his shouting at me and blaming me for our financial woes. I also didn't like Ri to hear the screaming and cursing that would come from his lips. I wanted to yell back at him and sometimes, due to complete exhaustion and utter frustration of living in the negative environment, I would yell at him. I hated what was happening. I never wanted to have an explosive marriage where the couples fight the majority of the time, yet this was exactly what was happening in the marriage. This was just another stressor to add to all of the other stressors in our lives.

The months dragged on and in 2008 I began to have to tap into our home equity line of credit to pay the mortgage, the property taxes, home insurance premium, all of the realtor fees, the medical co-pays and prescriptions, the utility bills and so on. Pat's income just didn't cover all of the living expenses that we had. The hospital co-pay for my total thyroidectomy was hundreds of dollars. A few weeks after my surgery we had another lean birthday party for Ri. I felt so guilty that I couldn't give her an amazing birthday bash like her other friends were having. I seemed to always feel guilty about something.

Then in the summer of 2008 we received a large check in the mail. It was Pat's inheritance from his mom, Carole. She lost her battle with lung cancer in February of 2007. We began to pay off credit card debts because we had been using credit cards to pay for our living and medical expenses. We still didn't have enough money to pay off the home equity line of credit. When Pat discovered that there wasn't enough money to pay that particularly large debt, he became furious and began to accuse me of stealing his mom's inheritance from him. He was vicious in his accusations verbally assaulting me and calling me vulgar names. All during our thirteen years of marriage I was very scared of these rages that he would go into. I felt defenseless because I was still recovering from my surgery, slowly, I might add. I felt humiliated and ashamed to be treated in such a fashion, especially by the very person who had promised to love, honor, and cherish me in sickness and health. I would literally have a sick feeling in the pit of my stomach when Pat would go into these rages. I felt powerless and disgusted all at the same time. Our lives were spinning out of control due to financial pressures.

By 2009 the financial pressures were gripping us like a mighty vise. Even though Pat worked full time as a cashier, was a realtor and had made three sales in the latter part of 2008 we still continued to come up short. It was approaching one year since my total thyroidectomy but I had a myriad of health issues that were making it impossible for me to work full-time. We discussed the possibility of me going to real estate school and although I didn't want to, I reluctantly agreed. The reason that I agreed is because I thought that giving into Pat's insistence that I become a realtor would stop him from going into these rages against me over the financial pressures we had. Of course I was wrong.

In February of 2009 I enrolled in a two-week real estate salesperson crash course. I took notes while both of my eyes continually teared (a Graves' disease symptom) and the instructor noticed I was having problems with my eyes and asked if I was okay. I was on a fast track to total stress burnout but I couldn't get off now so I just did the best that I could.

After passing the school national and state exams, I'll share that prior to successfully passing them, I failed the National Real Estate exam once and the State Real Estate exam twice. This devastated me because I was a college graduate and yet was struggling to pass these real estate exams. I spent hours of studying but I wasn't studying effectively. Much to my embarrassment I sat in on a couple of the classes over again before I went back to take the State exam the third time. It was on the third try that I successfully passed the State exam! After the proctor told me that I had passed the exam, I remember going into the bathroom at the testing center and literally sobbing for several minutes in thanks to God for finally passing the test.

Surely I thought this real estate accomplishment would please Pat because he had wanted me to become a realtor for years. I anticipated that he would now stop yelling at me, cursing at me, calling me filthy, vulgar names. As Ri and I were driving on the SR51 in my Saab 9 3 Convertible after leaving the AZ Dept of Real Estate, I felt that I was finally emerging out of life in the cave while listening to Jacki Velasquez sing "back into the light again". It was thrilling and exhilarating to feel that dark force growing dimmer and the light of hope and possibility becoming brighter as the wind whipped through our hair while we laughed and celebrated this important milestone.

That evening when Pat came home from work I excitedly told him I had passed the exam, drove straight over to the AZ Dept of Real Estate to get registered, then went to his broker's office to sign up and I was now officially an active realtor. I asked him if we could go out to eat to celebrate. He yelled at me, called me a (insert inappropriate slang term) and told me he had worked all day long and he was too tired to go out. After he spent a while on the computer he went to bed. I don't even remember what Ri and I ate for dinner that evening.

The months went by slowly. The first six months of 2009 brought no financial relief. We were talking about the real possibility of losing our house in foreclosure. The arguments became more volatile. Pat would curse at me, scream at me, accuse me of stealing his mom's inheritance when he woke up, when he came home from work and even in the middle of the night he would wake me up yelling at me and start the whole cycle over again the next morning. Finally, early in June of 2009, I could no longer mentally or emotionally handle his rage and anger. I filed for divorce and Ri and I went into hiding. During this time I was working on my Final Edits for *Life in the Cave Overcoming Graves' Disease* at the hotel where we hid during the summer. This helped me to not slip back into utter despair. It was a task I desperately needed as I continued to emerge from the cave.

Ri and I bonded even closer as we enjoyed swimming in the pool, took Jett (Ri's Norwegian Forest cat) for walks, and dined in the onsite restaurant. We would linger at our table by the fountain in the evenings and as we listened to the water flowing in the fountain it relaxed us and healed our hearts. It was in these quiet moments that I would meditate on "Be still and know that I am God." Ri and I would smile at each other as we both felt the presence of the Lord with us. His light was with us while we were in hiding. He was giving us hope for a brighter future.

The brightness came to us as we became fast friends with both waitresses Donna and Phyllis. They consistently were kind to Ri. I appreciated the way they affirmed Ri by including her in conversations. I believe that God brought these two beautiful women into our lives to bring us light as we hid at the hotel.

Although we were in hiding, this moment in time continued the process of emerging from the cave. Ri and I had a glimpse of what our lives could be like surrounded by people who respected us and genuinely enjoyed our company.

Chapter Eight
Relationships

My first endocrinologist, Dr. Dolinar, informed us that many married couples divorce when one of the spouses has Graves' disease. He went on to say that the personality of the Graves' disease patient dramatically alters and the healthy partner sometimes can't deal with all of the personality changes. All I can share is that I was very irritable and the financial pressures aggravated all of the negative forces a million times over. I just knew that I had to get Ri and I to a safe place before we began to be physically harmed; we were already emotionally and mentally abused by Pat. Ri was not directly abused but she still was a victim as she watched and listened in terror at the way her father was negatively treating her mother. Please keep in mind that we had a troubled marriage to begin with. If you are married it doesn't mean that you will wind up in divorce court. You need to be prepared to seek outside help, though, if serious problems arise that are not effectively resolved and you and your partner want to save your marriage.

By this time, the spring of 2009, I had no desire to reconcile with Pat. I didn't want to go to counseling. I didn't want to work on the marriage. I was done with this verbally abusive man who made me feel subhuman. I was a prisoner in my own home and I was very angry that I had stooped so low and unable to defend myself better. I was a college graduate, bright, talented and yet made to feel like the lowest of the lowest object on the planet. I hated Pat's behavior toward me and I hated myself for staying in this abusive relationship for so long. Back in the fall of 2001 I had planned to leave Pat and start a new life with my daughter. So once again, bear in mind, my marriage was troubled for nearly a decade before I finally filed for divorce and left in 2009.

This experience was another part of emerging from the cave. I slowly began to believe that I could remove from this subversive relationship in spite of the obstacles of not working full-time and battling an incurable disease. I welcomed this feeling of empowerment.

Your relationships with family, friends and the community are affected and normally change when you have Graves' disease. How close you are to family members, how often you see your friends and how active you are in the community will all yield different relationship results for every individual diagnosed with Graves' disease. The best you can do is to provide awareness and education for those you are in relationship with in an effort to help them understand that it is the Graves' disease that is causing your personality to alter reminding them to not take your irritability personally. A suggestion would be for them to leave the area for a while and do a pleasant activity from you when they can tell you are in a particularly foul mood. This gives you the space you need to get over it and the opportunity they need to refuel as well.

I strongly urge you to not try to go it alone if you have Graves' disease. You need people in your life that sincerely love you and care about your wellbeing. You need to know that you are loved. You need that hug. You need that word of encouragement. You need to know that you matter. I appreciated the phone calls from my mom, my sister, and my brothers. My mom and sister also sent me thoughtful cards to brighten my days.

Open communication is what will save you in your relationships. You may want to consider individual counseling and family counseling if there are unhealthy ways of dealing with stress present in your closest of relationships. If you're still able to work I would suggest scheduling a meeting with your employer. It may be helpful to bring along Graves' disease articles to share that may help facilitate dialogue, education, empathy and understanding from your employer. Further, if your endocrinologist is open and available, ask if he/she would be willing to discuss Graves' disease with your employer providing an opportunity to gain knowledge about this disease from a medical professional.

You are in control of your relationships more than you realize. Even the best of relationships experience the ebb and flow of life and you need these meaningful relationships to get you through the dark days. An effective way to deal with your irritability and frustration is to journal those negative feelings you are experiencing in your relationships with others. Write them down. Read them. Vent them on paper. Then allow forgiveness to come from deep inside you for the offense and allow your love for that person to flow once again. Remember the ebb and flow and remind yourself of what drew you to that wonderful person in the first place.

You are forever changed and once you can accept that fact you will feel more empowered as you interact with others. Remember it is up to you to educate and stoke Graves' disease awareness in your relationships. Just as they need to be patient with you it is wise to remember that you need to be patient with them. You have changed and it will take time to adjust to these personality changes on everyone's part.

I challenge you to turn this deficit of irritability into an asset. You can do it. It will take effort and endurance while you all work through the necessary adjustments in your changed relationships. Don't give up, though. You will make it to the other side and look back to see how much closer and tighter your bonds are in these special relationships in your life. The joy that I've experienced in my relationships has continued the process of emerging from the cave and the light shines brighter each day. As far as relationships in the community it varies for each person. Some of you may have been very active in your community and I challenge you to become a Graves' disease awareness activist in your circle of influence. There is a need for the world to know that Graves' disease is an autoimmune disorder that there is no cure for. It is a real disease with grave (no pun intended) results, for example, thyroid storm, where body temperature, blood pressure and heart rate all go sky-high, is life-threatening and could result in a stroke or heart attack if not treated properly. The patient must immediately go to the hospital to receive proper treatment for thyroid storm symptoms. Most people have never heard of Graves' disease. Let's change that fact and become the voice for those who have just been diagnosed and are too afraid, fatigued, overwhelmed and stressed to share their stories of their battle with Graves' disease. Let's be their voice until they are strong enough to speak up.

I have had family members, former coworkers, college friends and friends I've lost contact with over the years read my first book, *Life in the Cave Overcoming Graves' Disease* and call me (some even write to me) to apologize, even cry, because they weren't there for me. I don't have any ill will or grudges with these amazing people who have shaped my life. How could I when I didn't even understand what was happening to me before I was diagnosed? I do know that I now have an obligation to educate folks on Graves' disease as I've become stronger and am surviving Graves' disease.

In your relationships it is important to feel safe and also comforting to know you have support in these meaningful relationships. Support is key to surviving Graves' disease and the last chapter will explore this important topic.

Chapter Nine
Support

In closing, you must have support. Even if all you have is the support of one other person on the planet consider yourself rich. You cannot, I repeat, you cannot survive Graves' disease on your own. You need the support of others. A reader shared with me how she loved the title of my book *Life in the Cave* because that is exactly how she felt, like she was in a cave. It is so easy to believe the lie that you are on your own, that no one understands, that no one cares. Well, dear reader. I care. Folks who are members of and/or associated with the National Graves' Disease and Thyroid Foundation care, too. You are not alone. Even though only a small amount of the population has been diagnosed with Graves' disease each of us knows what it is like to feel overwhelmed with the many facets of Graves' disease and we are eager to stoke Graves' disease awareness.

In Chapter Eight, I shared the importance of support in our relationships. Now I'd like to take a moment to look at online and local support groups.

There are many online Graves' disease discussion boards out in cyberspace. If you are a member of Facebook, I personally invite you to "like" my Life in the Cave Overcoming Graves' Disease Series facebook page located at https://www.facebook.com/LifeInTheCave

There are other Graves' disease support groups and pages on Facebook, too. Another great place to go for online support, and in my opinion one of the best online resources, is https://www.gdatf.org

The National Graves' Disease and Thyroid Foundation has support groups in many states throughout the United States and in Canada. They are actively adding new support groups, too. Even if your state doesn't have a support group now the chances are good that it will eventually have one.

Lastly, I warmly invite you to email me at celiamariellc@gmail.com as I would love to hear your story. Please know that you are not alone in your battle with Graves' disease. I read each e-mail and personally answer every e-mail. Sometimes I do get behind on e-mails but I assure you that at some point you will hear directly from me.

Thank you for reading my story. It has been difficult to share some of the most intimate details of my life here with you but if it can help in some small way to aid you in surviving Graves' disease then it has been worth it.

BOOK THREE

Beyond Graves' Disease: Thoughts and Reflections

Beyond Graves' Disease
Thoughts and Reflections

CELIA MARIE

Celia Marie, LLC
2020

Published in the United States of America
ISBN: 978-0-557-40914-3
1. Health & Fitness/Diseases/Immune System
2. Health & Fitness/Diseases/General

I dedicate this book to all who have been diagnosed with Graves' disease. I challenge each of you to become an over comer of Graves' disease, moving Beyond Graves' and on to the endless possibilities that await you now that you have been forever changed. Share your stories and raise Graves' disease awareness. I salute you.

Acknowledgements

Ri, you have my deepest gratitude. I could have never made it without you. You have been there every step of the way, at every doctor's visit (there've been hundreds), every medical procedure, at the hospital during my surgery and at home. Your constant reminder of "I love you" on a daily basis pushed me when I was fed up with the battle. Your continual forgiveness each time I have blown it with you has been the fragrance that has made the most difficult times bearable. Ri, you have an amazing amount of compassion, cheerfulness and patience. I pray that you will always remember the time you told me "Mom, what this world needs the most is Jesus." Ri, you are God's mouthpiece in your generation. I am thankful that you were given to me as a gift from God. Continue to share your light and infectious laughter with the world!

I am thankful to Pat for providing the much needed medical insurance, paying for the co-pays and prescriptions. Thank you.

Thank you, Glynis. Your daily prayers, encouragement, phone calls, cards with a little something extra, all of the laughter, in addition to you listening to my heart more than my words has all been part of this journey. By the time this book releases we will have been friends for 25 years! I am amazed at how God could bring two women together who are so different and yet knitted together so closely; of course this goes much deeper than our mutual appreciation of "It's a Mad, Mad, Mad, Mad World" and "Anne of Green Gables." I love you, Glynis.

Introduction

August 2008

As I sat in the auditorium at Vineyard Church North Phoenix in August of 2008, I looked around at the congregation. My mind was wandering (which is not uncommon when you have Graves' disease) and then I looked back at Pastor Brian T. Anderson as I focused in on the words coming from his lips. "Your life is a book," he said, "you are the one who must decide if your book is going to be a good one or a great one."

For weeks my friend, Glynis, and I had been talking about the book I was planning to write. It all started out as a joke. One day I was pouring my heart out to her on the phone and I jokingly said that I should write a book about all of this and she bantered back that it would be on the bestseller list. Even though we talked about my book several times since that conversation I began to ponder if that is what I was supposed to do. What if I was supposed to write about my journey with Graves' disease?

I had been involved in journalism since my junior high days. In senior high school I was a member of the Quill and Scroll Society, co-editor of our school newspaper, feature editor of same newspaper and after I graduated from college I began my 501C-3 called Pure Stoke Press. I wrote and published articles for extreme sports enthusiasts on topics of surfing, running, hiking, and skiing. My article "Climb the Mountain" was distributed at the annual Walk for Cancer at South Mountain in Phoenix, Arizona. My "Pure Stoke" article (for surfers) was given to surfers at Imperial Beach, Tourmaline Surfing Park and even found its' way to Hawaii. I also wrote an article on the Iditarod that was handed out at the Kuskokwim 300 dog sled race in Bethel, Alaska. As my mind once again focused on the words that Pastor Anderson was speaking he said "In closing, it's up to you to decide if your life is going to be a good book or a great book." I began to think that I was not only supposed to write just one book, but a trilogy of my journey with Graves' disease. As the service was ending I prayed that if this was the path that God wanted me to take that He would let me know and give me the words to write.

May 2010

The book you are about to read is the third book in my Graves' disease series. Part of me is hesitating to begin writing the first chapter because I know that this will be my last book in this series while another part of me is thrilled to begin writing this book. Many of you have read my books, *Life in the Cave Overcoming Graves' Disease* and *Emerging From the Cave Surviving Graves' Disease*. Both of them focus on not only how Graves' disease has affected me but how it has also affected my family and friends.

My purpose in writing Beyond Graves' Disease is to share idioms, quotes and verses that have become meaningful to me upon discovering that I have Graves' disease which is treatable but not curable. My life has been forever changed. I have chosen to not give up but to go on. This choice was not easy. From the years 2005-2008 I bitterly fought all of the symptoms, went through the denial, the paralysis of fear, the deep pain, sorrow, and anger; yet, before my surgery there was a turning point where I made a conscious decision to choose to live and to not let the fear of living with Graves' disease rob me of a beautiful life filled with each new day of the wonder of the possibilities that lie ahead. I chose to live for my daughter's sake but what I've received is far much more than any expectations I had dreamed of and hoped for. The words that you are about to read are vignettes of possibility, hope, light, dreams, laughter and surrender. I offer you the words of someone who doesn't dream it's over. Limitless possibilities are my focus now.

1.

Never give in. Never give in. Never, never, never, never – in nothing, great or small, large or petty—never give in, except to convictions of honor and good sense.
Winston Churchill

Many times I was tempted to give up during my battle with Graves' disease. Each time I was tempted to throw in the towel I would remember these wise words of Winston Churchill.

2.

Rome wasn't built in a day.

French Proverb

I really love this proverb because it reminds me to be gentle with myself. The important things in life take time. Your healing recovery may come in a split second but mine has been in the making for four years.

3.

> *"The LORD your God in your midst, The Mighty One, will save; He will rejoice over you with gladness, He will quiet you with His love, He will rejoice over you with singing."*
>
> Zepheniah 3:17

This verse became very special to me in September of 2009. During one of my daily devotions the Lord impressed upon me through my cognitive processes that although I was experiencing deep sorrow He was going to give me a new song (Psalm 40:3). I immediately thought of the above verse taking great comfort and immense joy in the promise that He is saving me, rejoicing in me, His creation, with singing! This is very beautiful and precious to me that the Creator of the universe takes notice and delights in me. I am complete in this all-encompassing affirmation of my Heavenly Father.

Be God's
Rich Mullins

This one is a challenge and my heart's deepest desire. I want to "**Be God's**" yet in order to truly do this I must choose to die to myself many times in the course of a day. If I am to be His I need to let go of my wants, wishes, and desires to be the vessel that He can use and flow through.

It is a very frightening thing to let go to "**Be God's**". If you choose to do this please e-mail me at CeliaMarieLLC@gmail.com and share your experience of how you've accepted Rich Mullins challenge to "**Be God's**". I also welcome hearing from you if you are a fan of Rich Mullins. His songs are truly the soundtrack of my life.

5.

An apple a day keeps the doctor away.
Ancient Roman Proverb

The naturopathic approach to healing includes healthy eating. Apples are a source of Vitamin C which is good for our immune system. They also contain fiber and bioflavonoids

6.

A merry heart does good, like medicine,
But a broken spirit dries the bones.
Proverbs 17:22

Laughter is conducive to healing. Surround yourself around positive people. Go watch a comedy. Read a humorous book. Laugh at yourself. Listen to upbeat music with a positive message. Laugh at yourself. Yes, I repeated that on purpose!

For I know the thoughts that I think toward you, says the LORD, thoughts of peace and not of evil, to give you a future and a hope.
Jeremiah 29:11

This is truly my life verse. I chose this while I was in college. I trust this promise completely. Do you have a life verse? Please e-mail me at <u>CeliaMarieLLC@gmail.com</u> and share your life verse with me.

8.

Birds of a feather flock together.
16th Century Proverb

This is so true. Do you want peace in your life? Do you want Truth in your life? Do you want laughter in your life? Do you want stimulating conversation in your life? Seek peaceful, truthful, humorous, interesting people to spend your time with.

9.

And you shall know the truth, and the truth
shall make you free.

John 8:32

It takes courage to seek the truth. When I was 33 I was on a serious quest for truth. I meant business and this quest took me to sitting in a chair across from Ellen, my counselor. She saw me weekly in the beginning because I was so distraught. She explained to me that my cup had overflowed and that was why I found a need to meet with her. She went on to say that she wished that victims like me would not be bound in the shame of what they had survived. She told me the truth. The truth was what happened to me was not my fault. She showed me that my abusers were affected by what they had done to me just as much as I was affected. Week after week, month after month we peeled back the layers of shame, humiliation, grief, and deep pain: gradually while we were stripping away every deception I was becoming a young woman experiencing true freedom for the very first time. Thank you, Ellen, and thank you God. I feel compelled to share that this verse literally means that Jesus Christ is the Truth and He truly makes us free. Through Jesus we have redemption and resurrection because He was wounded for our transgressions and by His stripes we are healed of any physical, spiritual, emotional or mental affliction we are either battling or have been freed of. He is God's gift of love to the world and whoever believes and accepts His son, Jesus Christ, as their personal Savior will have everlasting life.

10.

*Forgiveness is the fragrance that the violet
sheds on the heel that has crushed it.*

Mark Twain

There is power, strength and beauty in forgiveness. Do
you need to forgive someone today? Let the powerful healing
of forgiveness set you free.

11.

Nothing great was ever achieved without enthusiasm.
Ralph Waldo Emerson

Think about your greatest achievements. Were you enthusiastic in your pursuit of your achievements? Your enthusiasm will realize great accomplishments.

12.

Follow your bliss.
Joseph Campbell

This is amazing. I have discovered that my God-given talents and abilities have led me straight to my bliss. I am thankful to God for the unique talents and abilities that He's given to me.

Yet in all these things we are more than conquerors through Him who loved us. For I am persuaded that neither death nor life, nor angels nor principalities, nor powers, nor things present nor things to come, nor height nor depth, nor any other created thing, shall be able to separate us from the love of God which is in Christ Jesus our Lord.

Romans 8:37-39

This promise has sustained me through the most difficult times of my life. I believe in this passage and know that this Truth has helped in my journey of healing with Graves' disease. I am not fully healed and there is no cure for Graves' disease but I have come so far in comparison to where I was when first diagnosed with Graves' disease in September of 2006.

14.

> *The Lord bless you and keep you; the Lord*
> *make His face shine upon you, and be gracious to*
> *you; the Lord lift up His countenance upon you,*
> *And give you peace.*
> Numbers 6:24-26

This blessing is my favorite. I look forward to Pastor Brian T. Anderson speaking this over our congregation. I soak in the peace, comfort and joy that these words bring to give me nourishment for the coming week.

Epilogue

June 2010

The 14 idioms, quotes and verses that I have shared with you all have special meaning to me. Of course I have many more but these stand out to me the most at this time in my life.

I thank you for joining me as I have shared my journey with Graves' disease in my books, *Life in the Cave Overcoming Graves' Disease, Emerging from the Cave Surviving Graves' Disease* and this book you're now holding in your hands *Beyond Graves' Disease Thoughts and Reflections.* I chose to not put my whole focus on the negative aspect of Graves' disease in this book because my perspective on my life at this point in the journey is recovery. I believe that we each have four components in our being, physical, spiritual, emotional and mental. I wanted to touch on each aspect within these pages. In order to be in balance we need to nurture each of these areas.

Further, I have surrendered my old life in exchange for my new life. I look forward to watching Ri, my daughter, carve out her own life with all our future moments of laughter, joy, hugs, failures, heart-to-heart talks, prayers, disagreements, misunderstandings and forgiveness that are on the horizon. I am excited about the plans that the Lord has for me and Ri.

My newest hobby is learning new languages. I also continue to enjoy social media sites including Facebook and Myspace.

I have discovered that my bliss is now the field of screenwriting. I am looking forward to this new chapter in my life as a screenwriter. I believe that we need quality films that focus on integrity, justice, education and faith. I would love to offer a quality film educating the public about Graves' disease.

I wish you the best in your journey with Graves' disease or any other disease from which you are recovering. Please e-mail me at CeliaMarieLLC@gmail.com and share your story of recovery with me. I would love to hear from you.

AFTERWARD

May 2020

In closing, the past decade has been a journey that has had many bends, curves, stops, starts, uphill and downhill moments as I've walked through, up, over the hills and down in the valleys while adjusting to a new "normal". It has been a journey I'll never forget. Thank you for allowing me to share my journey with you in my *Life in the Cave: The Series* book.

I look forward to the day when a cure will be found for Graves' disease. Until then, please remember that you are not alone. We are overcoming this insidious autoimmune disease together. We are working towards limitless possibilities each day. It's a beautiful day to raise Grave's disease awareness.